CPD in the Built Environment

The aim of this book is to provide a single source of information to support continuing professional development (CPD) in the built environment sector.

The book offers a comprehensive introduction to the concept of CPD and provides robust guidance on the methods and benefits of identifying, planning, monitoring, actioning, and recording CPD activities. It brings together theories, standards, professional and industry requirements, and contemporary arguments around individual personal and professional development. Practical techniques and real-life best practice examples outlined from within and outside of the industry empower the reader to take control of their own built environment-related development, whilst also providing information on how to develop fellow staff members. The contents covered in this book align with the requirements of numerous professional bodies, such as the Royal Institution of Chartered Surveyors, the Institution of Civil Engineers, and the Chartered Institute of Builders.

The chapters are supported by case studies, templates, practical advice, and guidance. The book is designed to help all current and future built environment professionals manage their own CPD as well as managing the CPD of others. This includes helping undergraduate and postgraduate students complete CPD requirements for modules as part of a wide range of built environment university degree courses and current built environment professionals of all levels and disciplines who wish to enhance their careers through personal and professional development, whether due to professional body requirements or by taking control of identifying and achieving their own educational needs.

Greg Watts is the Director of Quantity Surveying at the University of Salford and an RICS Chartered Quantity Surveyor with 15 years' experience in the construction industry and has published numerous conference and journal papers to date.

Norman Watts is a Senior Lecturer at Sheffield Hallam University and the Course Leader for MSc Construction Project Management. Norman has over 20 years' experience in teaching in Further and Higher Education and has publications in project management and quality systems.

CPD in the Built Environment

Greg Watts and Norman Watts

Routledge
Taylor & Francis Group
LONDON AND NEW YORK

First published 2021
by Routledge
2 Park Square, Milton Park, Abingdon, Oxon OX14 4RN

and by Routledge
52 Vanderbilt Avenue, New York, NY 10017

Routledge is an imprint of the Taylor & Francis Group, an informa business

British Library Cataloguing-in-Publication Data
A catalogue record for this book is available from the British Library

Library of Congress Cataloging-in-Publication Data
Names: Watts, Greg (Gregory N.), author. | Watts, Norman, author.
Title: CPD in the built environment / Greg Watts and Norman Watts.
Description: Abingdon, Oxon ; New York : Routledge/ Taylor & Francis Group, 2021. | Includes bibliographical references and index.
Identifiers: LCCN 2020048259 (print) | LCCN 2020048260 (ebook) | ISBN 9780367372149 (hardback) | ISBN 9780367372156 (paperback) | ISBN 9780429353062 (ebook)
Subjects: LCSH: Building—Study and teaching. | Building—Vocational guidance. | Continuing education.
Classification: LCC TH165 .W37 2021 (print) | LCC TH165 (ebook) | DDC 624.071/5—dc23
LC record available at https://lccn.loc.gov/2020048259
LC ebook record available at https://lccn.loc.gov/2020048260

ISBN: 978-0-367-37214-9 (hbk)
ISBN: 978-0-367-37215-6 (pbk)
ISBN: 978-0-429-35306-2 (ebk)

Typeset in Goudy
by codeMantra

Contents

Foreword

The construction industry is tasked with the development and maintenance of the built and natural environments. It covers areas of building, civil engineering, materials manufacture, and consultancy services contributing to and impacting upon the very fabric of our society. The industry contributes 6% of the total UK economic output and employs more than 2.4 million workers from over 340,000 businesses. However, the construction industry faces a serious predicament and is in need of change.

This change is driven by a shrinking traditional workforce, technology advancements, and the increasing imperative for sustainable solutions. For some, this change is not fast enough. Many professional and industry leading bodies, as well as significant industry reports, have called for change across many fronts. Such changes have included the need to adopt modern construction methods, embrace innovative and disruptive technologies, collaborate across supply chain disciplines, implement sustainability strategies, overcome adversarial attitudes, and improve the industry's core productivity problem. Arguably underpinning all of these challenges is the need for the construction industry to develop its workforce.

The development of technical and professional skill sets and competencies ultimately takes the form of continuing professional development (CPD). Simply put, CPD refers to the identification of required skills, competencies and experience, identification of gaps in the current knowledge, setting goals to address these gaps, and the undertaking of planned activities required to achieve those goals before finally reflecting upon the process. It is only through effective individual and industry-wide CPD that professionals can understand the current and future needs of the built environment and help drive the changes the construction industry requires.

With their combination of construction industry and academic experience, the authors are well placed to address the gap in CPD guidance that currently exists in the industry, with *CPD in the Built Environment* serving to offer a comprehensive introduction to, and application of, CPD. This textbook provides guidance to all professionals operating within the built environment on how effective CPD can be undertaken and managed.

Mark Farmer
CEO Cast Consultancy & UK Government MMC
Champion for Homebuilding

Preface

The construction industry is changing. For some, this change is not happening fast enough nor going far enough. There have been an increasing number of industry leading reports published with each calling for change in the construction industry. This change ranges from the adoption of innovative practices to the modernisation of construction methods and from the need for increased collaboration across all stakeholders to a desire to focus on more value-led approaches. Underlining all these calls for change and the actions required to enact such changes is the need for the continuing professional development (CPD) of all construction industry professionals.

The aim of this book is to provide CPD guidance for all professionals operating at every level of the built environment and for those wanting to work in the built environment and studying on related courses. When enacted correctly, CPD plays a pivotal role in the development of skills and progression of careers. This book emphasises the increasing importance of CPD and attempts to equip readers with the skills and knowledge to create effective CPD plans and the methods of effectively managing the CPD plans of others. Hopefully this book serves this purpose and is enjoyable and informative to read.

Greg Watts
Norman Watts

Acknowledgements

For Anna. Your support helped make this book happen. Greg

Dedicated to Julie Heather. Norman

1 What is continuing professional development?

1.1 Introduction

The intention of this chapter is to offer the reader a useful starting point to understanding the significance that continuing professional development (CPD) plays in the career of the construction professional. Contemporary issues in construction professional development within the built environment are explored, and the benefits as advocated by professional institutions and organisations are identified. Key stages of CPD are shown and approaches to CPD activities provide useful primer to those readers wishing to use CPD in the development of their own career path. Mentoring and peer learning is highlighted as a helpful tool for identifying skills gaps and gaining knowledge. Critical thinking is identified as one of the key pivotal elements needed when determining the appropriate professional development needs.

1.1.1 History of continuing professional development

CPD, or as it is sometimes called continuing professional development, has its roots in the term 'professional development' which relates to a person's work. Professionals such as senior managers, doctors, teachers, and legal experts all take part in professional development activities in order to apply these newfound skills and knowledge in their place of work that will contribute to improved performance.

Research and development in the field of professional development has been around for over 150 years and focused mainly in the education sectors. The term 'continuous improvement' gained prominence in post-war 1950s which saw the reconstruction of large economies such as the likes of Japan's automotive manufacturer Toyota. The company implement a concept known as 'Kaizen' in its production process. The meaning of Kaizen is 'improvement' or 'continuously improve'. Known as continual improvement process (CIP), this is an ongoing iterative effort to improve the system or process for an improved product or service.

The 1960s–1980s saw steps in the development of organisation implementing training/learning and professional development. Authors such as W.E. Deeming on Quality System in manufacturing processes and other research reports, for example, from the construction sector such as 'Continuing professional development for Architects: Report on a research study' by Richard Gardner et al. (1981) brought the concept of CPD to most professions.

CPD much like Kaizen's link to CIP embraces in-service or on-the-job training beyond any baseline training initially expected to carry out a job role. In quality systems, feedback for process improvement would help enhance the system much like the case of professional improvement; reflective feedback would help to improve ways of working.

Simply put modern CPD refers to the identification of a skills/experience or knowledge gap in one's profession, recording the training activity after the event and reflecting on its application. An activity log is kept and continually update as required. CPD is a process and will continue throughout the one's career and supports lifelong learning.

The key steps are as follows:

1 Identify the gap in your knowledge, skills, or experience.
2 Find and attend a course or activity that will fill the gap.
3 Record the event.
4 Apply the knowledge, skills, or experience gained.
5 Reflect on the learning and development.
6 Repeat.

As with quality systems feedback (reflection) feeds back into to step 1 to start the continuous improvement process again.

A point to note here is regarding step 4 'apply the knowledge'. If you are unable to apply what has been learnt, then the previous three steps will have been a waste of time and money for you and, if paid for by your employers, the organisation.

To illustrate why step 4 is so critical, consider this anecdote:

> A Building Surveyor may identify a gap in knowledge in understanding Sustainable Draining Systems (SUDS) a more environmentally friendly approach to managing drainage in and around properties. The surveyor identifies a 2 day course, enrols, and completes it gaining a successful completion certificate. As a member of the Royal Institution of Chartered Surveyors, the surveyor records the event in their RICS CPD log. However, the surveyor does not get the chance to use this new knowledge in any future work. You could reasonably conclude then that this event has been a waste of time for the surveyor and the knowledge had no tangible merit in their professional development.
>
> However, on further reflection the course could have had merit in some other less-tangible way such as team building skills if the course happened to have used working in teams as part of the course delivery mechanism.

Subsequently for step 4 the surveyor could apply the knowledge, skill gained on the course it just happened to be in teambuilding on a challenging new project not in using SUDS knowledge.

It is important to recognise in step 1 that there must be a genuine need to fill a gap in knowledge and for improvement to occur, not simply improvement for improvements sake or attending a course for attendance sake.

1.2 Benefits to the practitioner

For the professional practitioner, benefits include career progression and advancement. This can usually be evidenced in their CV and expanded upon in any subsequent promotion interviews demonstrating their dedication to professional development.

The aim of most professional practitioners is to get chartered membership of an appropriate institution. Construction- and engineering-related institutions such as the Institution of Civil Engineers (ICE), the Royal Institution of Chartered Surveyors (RICS), the Royal Institute of British Architects (RIBA), and the Chartered Institute of Builders (CIOB) advocate the benefits for their members. A summary of these can be found in Table 1.1.

The Chartered Institute of Personnel Development provides a holistic view to the benefits of CPD and suggests that it "is an investment that you make in yourself". It goes on to confirm that the benefits can improve an individual's confidence as well as strengthening their professional credibility.

Table 1.1 Professional development benefits

• A way to show you are keeping your skills, knowledge, and experience up to date • Supports you to work safely, legally, and effectively • Career development • Shows commitment to lifelong learning • Demonstrates professional pride	• To remain professionally competent • To provide the best possible service • Considered a highly beneficial career tool • Can be used to strengthen the member's business skills • Can be used to acquire new skills	• Helps to stay competent, professional, and resilient as an architect • Helps to achieve better outcomes • Helps to achieve better businesses • Helps you contend with disruption • Helps to face current and future challenges • Helps to learn new skills and specialisms	• To be sure knowledge is up to date and complete • To stay professionally competent • To keep expertise up to scratch

1.3 Benefits to the client–customer

It is not unreasonable to suggest that clients and customers to the construction industry must have the confidence in the ability of the service provider. The expectation to have a project delivered on time to the right quality and at the agreed price forms the basis to any contract or agreement. Consequently, the relationship between the actual client or client's representative and the service provider's representative is often seen as the most important aspect of such an agreement.

The representative for the delivery organisation would typically be the Architect, Senior Quantity Surveyor, Construction Project Manager, or other designated professional.

Key to the purpose of the professional is to provide trust that a client, customer, or the public will receive a quality service. Education and training through CPD activities provides a higher level professionalism especially when the individual is part of a professional body such as RIBA. The professional body's role serves to maintain standards, ethics, and behaviours of its members as such, these professional bodies place CPD at the heart their approach to professional development by requiring their members to stay up to date with best practice standards. Construction clients and customers are likely to consider professionals who are members of chartered institutions more highly. The relationship between the professional and the institution is evident in respect to ethical standards maintained through ongoing training practices.

1.4 Benefits to the organisation

Many organisations see staff development as an integral part of their corporate social responsibility to their employees and will apportion a staff development budget to training programmes. The advocated benefits of CPD for staff and workforce include the following:

- It promotes staff development and ensures high standards across the organisation.
- It creates higher level of morale and retention when staff feel valued.
- It helps build a well-motivated workforce which is more likely to embrace change.
- It contributes to an organisation's growth and helps meet key organisational objectives.
- It improves productivity and the firm's competitiveness and profitability.

The aim of an organisation is to ensure that its employees are of a higher calibre and remain proficient in their role throughout their career not only by keeping up to date with knowledge, skills, and training but also by becoming Chartered members of recognised institutions.

Balfour Beatty, the largest construction company in the UK by turnover, states that "*The growth of our people is absolutely vital to our business. The better they are, the better we are...*" It goes on to advocate a layered approach to professional development, which includes the following:

- Controlling your career: encouraged to take personal control of your career.
- 70-20-10: approach to development – 70% on the job, 20% learning from those around you, and 10% formal training courses and learning events.
- Ongoing development: learning and development needs will be a key part of your performance review.
- Getting qualified: support to gain membership of a relevant professional institution.
- Brilliant basics: free modules for developing skills that are considered the foundation for success in every job.
- Learning to lead: programmes in everything from emotional intelligence to inclusive leadership.
- Taking the step up: through clear pathways for internal progression, always look to appoint from within.

This approach advocated by the organisation shows benefits between the success of the individual through personal development and the success of the company.

Further, the value of mentoring programmes in respect to an organisation's employee development strategy is well evidenced in research, concluding that organisations with structured programmes have better employee engagement and higher retention rates.

1.5 Approaches to CPD

As we now understand, CPD activities are undertaken by professionals to improve their occupational skills and knowledge. Broadly, any activity from which you can learn from or develop professionally can be considered as a CPD activity. Most common activities include: the following

- Conferences

  Conferences can often last a few days and tend to be themed around a topical academic or business matter. For example, a conference on Building Information Modelling will bring experts, industry practitioners, and those with an interest in the topic together.
- Seminars/talks

  Seminars and talks can last for a few hours and will be led by an expert on the subject matter and where the audience will have requested a place to attend specifically to acquire some subject knowledge. Often the seminar will end with the issuing of a CPD certificate of attendance to all attendees.
- Peer review

  Peer reviews are reviews of research articles or reports made by academics and sometimes industry practitioners. These reports are submitted to journals for publication or conference proceedings. Prior to acceptance the articles are 'peer reviewed' sent to other academics in the same field in order to assert validity in the subject field.

- Bespoke workshops

  Workshops tend to be a more interactive type of meeting attended by people to engage in acquiring new knowledge or a new skill in a specific area previously identified usually by senior management in an organisation. A workshop is set up to meet some training requirement.
- Courses (accredited/non-accredited)

  Courses are fixed programmes on individual subjects and delivered by expert tutors. These can last a few weeks or a few years for a university degree course. Sessions within the course will be a weekly event and will lead up to the submission of an assessment report or the sitting of an exam to test what the student has learnt and has met the course aims. Certificates are awarded on passing the course. An accredited course is subject to quality control from an independent professional body and as such is highly regarded by the industry. A non-accredited course is not subject to the same scrutiny so it may not be as well received by the industry. However, the student can still acquire the necessary knowledge and skills from non-accredited courses.
- Self-study

  Also known as self-directed learning, self-study is a learning method directed and paced by the learner. There is no direct supervision and is not set in a classroom. The learner takes full control of their own studying. Modern methods tend to be accessing online material and can learn at their own pace. Reading books and articles also support self-study.
- Graduate training programmes

  Several of the medium to large construction sector companies in the UK often run graduate training programmes, also known as graduate schemes. These schemes are typically entry-level posts with an employer who allows the graduate the opportunity to work in rotation across different departments in the company in order to gain knowledge and experience. A normal duration for a graduate scheme is no more than two years before the employer and employee agree the specific job role. Internal training will form part of the scheme and may include external CPD activities. Graduate programmes are offered to those students who have completed their university studies and are ready to enter full-time work.

When choosing any type of CPD activity it is worthwhile considering there is no one universal method that guarantees success in learning, mixing types are always worthwhile in order to learn from different delivery modes as this will broaden your experiences.

Institutions such as Chartered Institute of Professional Development (CIPD) offer a useful set of principles supporting CPD and lifelong learning. The institution's members are made of human resource and people development professionals from all industries and business sectors including the construction sector organisations and Higher Education. Table 1.2 shows the authors view of the CIPD's essential CPD principles.

These advocated principles are intended to allow for its chartered members to demonstrate their commitment to professionalism and commitment to CPD.

Table 1.2 The authors view of the CIPD's essential CPD principles

C – Continuing	• Members demonstrate a commitment to developing competence through the virtuous circle of CPD. • Development is continuous. Members actively seek to improve their knowledge, skills, and performance. • Regular investment of time and learning is seen as an essential part of professional life and not an optional extra.
P – Professional	• Members take an active interest in the internal and external environments and in the continuous development and improvement of self and others at both organisation and individual levels. • Learning objectives should be clear, serving individual, client and organisational needs.
D – Development	• The starting point is a realistic assessment of what needs to be learnt to meet the demands of the evolving professional and business worlds. • The individual takes responsibility for their development, learning from all experiences, combined with reflection as key activities. • Working effectively and inclusively with colleagues, clients, stakeholders, customers, teams and individuals both within and outside of the organisation.

Adapted from: https://www.cipd.co.uk/learn/cpd/policy.

Construction-related professional bodies also provide useful definitions, some short and punchy such as the RICS. "...*a commitment by RICS members to continually update their skills and knowledge in order to remain professionally competent*" (rics.org), although underpinning this is a more detailed compliance guide. The process includes documenting all CPD activities with some form of written review and reflection on lessons/knowledge learnt.

Professional practitioners who embark on a career in the construction sector see CPD as a means to becoming and staying a Chartered member. There are demonstrable benefits to the individual, to the organisation, and to the overall image of the sector.

1.6 Contemporary approaches to CPD

Other approaches to CPD learning used together with those traditional types mentioned above include the following:

1.6.1 Peer learning

Peer learning-based approaches can be as simple as a group of likeminded construction professionals holding regular formal or informal meetings to support, validate, and share their own achievements in learning by:

- Discussing and share learning experiences
- Reflecting on aspects best practice in their role

- Collaborating on specific difficult areas of challenges in the workplace
- Sharing personal learning achievements

As most construction-related professional institutions require CPD evidenced and measured essentially by the numbers of hours attended per year, some contemporary approaches can be difficult to quantify. However, it is important to recognise that these types of contemporary approaches can still support and enhance the individuals. Likewise, traditional CPD activities will also support the individuals and satisfy professional institution requirements.

Other peer learning models include but not limited to:

- Buddy systems: In the workplace, an experienced member of staff known as a 'buddy' will be assigned to an employee or new employee to guide and share knowledge. Sometimes both 'buddies' can be individuals teamed up to work together and help each other.
- Peer assessment schemes: Allow for individuals within a peer group to assess their own position or contribution to an activity and for others in the group to 'peer review' the individuals. Advocated outputs and learning in peer assessment schemes include goal setting, reflection, and contributions in collaborative efforts.
- Collaborative projects: Allow individuals to work collaboratively with other professionals in order to increase their application of knowledge in relation to their professional domain. Advocated benefits to collaboration are promoting team working and effective communication.

Peer learning is not a single strategy for learning, but it covers a broad range of activities which can often overlap. Peer teaching can be used when those with a little more experience help and instruct others; the role has a similar function as a mentor.

1.6.2 Mentoring

For the seasoned built environment professional such as senior quantity surveyor or construction project manager, taking on and supporting junior members of the team and helping them to learn can be a rewarding experience for both. For the mentor it is an opportunity to share in the experiences gained and life lessons learnt over a professional career. Mentoring also offers several benefits for the mentee (the person being mentored). These include the following:

- Improved job performance
- Enhanced job satisfaction
- Deeper commitment to the organisation
- Improved problem-solving skills

Mentoring helps support the mentee's professional development, and it has to be a relationship that is based upon mutual respect for it to work effectively. It is not normally the role of the mentor to teach, but to listen, encourage, be a critical friend, and where appropriate point the mentee in the right direction. Chapter 8 explores the role played by mentoring in more detail.

Formal mentoring programmes within an organisation can facilitate career opportunities for employees and often enable a more positive culture in the workplace. Structured mentoring programmes are often a function of Human Resources and will frequently take the form of:

- Peer mentoring: It takes place between two people who may share the same job title. One will have the experience and knowledge of the role and will help and support the person new to the role.
- Group mentoring: It works in a group or team setting. The individual being mentored will have the opportunity to learn from a group of experts. Group mentoring can often include more than one learner (mentee).
- Reverse mentoring: It is offered to senior members of the organisation and mentored, for example, by junior recruits. It is designed to help senior staff to stay relevant and understand new and fresh ideas such as cultural relevance. In some instances, reverse mentoring has been used to "equip senior leaders with the skills needed to embed an inclusive culture withing teams" (balfourbeatty.com) in order to share insights into the experience of ethnic minorities and other underrepresented groups.

Mentoring programmes offer a structured approach to career development and will often include a pool of mentors from the organisation who are prepared to help and support career-minded individuals.

1.6.3 Critical thinking

Critical thinking can be viewed as the ability to think rationally in a clear unobstructed way about events and ideas. The ability to critical think allows for an optimum solution to be arrived at or an understanding to be gained of a past or present event. Critical thinking on past events will likely sit within the area of 'critical reflection' as both share the same analytical skills. Critical thinking and critical reflection are often interwoven, and Chapter 6 explores critical reflection in more detail.

A critical thinker will take an active approach to learning and understanding; this itself requires learning. So, learning how to learn is learning how to critically think in order to learn. Skills of the critical thinker include the following:

- Having a systematic approach to problem-solving
- Having the ability to distinguish between relevant and irrelevant
- Recognising interconnections between ideas
- Articulating and justifying decisions made or solutions arrived at
- Recognising own limitations and its influence on decisions made

The last point offers a useful insight for those who consider themselves to be a critical thinker. Critical thinking is not a 24/7 process; emotions can often determine an incorrect course of action or solution. Thinking critically allows the individual to differentiate between what is subject or emotional and what is objective or rational. Understanding this helps the learner towards being a better critical thinker which takes a few years of practice.

For the construction professional, critical thinking skills will help recognise the appropriate professional development needs and identify the short-term learning requirements to achieve the long-term goals.

Activities for improving critical thinking include the following:

- Reviewing a book/film/academic paper
- Recognising fake news and distinguishing between what is truthful and what is misleading
- Delivering seminars to peers
- Writing an essay
- Reflecting on a previous project and identifying what went right and what did not go right
- Presenting your findings to the project team

All the above have one thing in common: they challenge you to think about a situation more objectively. However, critical thinking can be a difficult goal to achieve and take determination and require focus. Take routine work tasks for example; these do not require any degree of higher level thinking as these are everyday occurrences that you understand and instinctively do. Where you are in situations that are not routine and require a new approach or a distinctive solution, you are faced with the need to think more critically in order to achieve the desired outcomes. This higher level thinking also applies to professional development and helps in choosing the correct CPD activities. Thinking critically about your development goals and gaps in your skills or knowledge allows for appropriate decision-making strategies to be employed. Thinking critically on CPD helps when:

- Justifying a course of action or decision
- Aligning CPD activities towards career goals
- Demonstrating critical reflection

For CPD, critical thinking can be best viewed as an evaluation technique for supporting decision-making on how to meet some pre-defined goals. Higher level senior managers will tend to have learnt critical thinking skills through their career progression. It is not a skill gained overnight, but it will have taken many attempts, mistakes, and realisations. The relationship between critical thinking, professional development, and CPD demonstrates its importance to the construction professional in the built environment.

1.7 Conclusion

The term 'CPD', as most companies and professional practitioners know of it today, has its roots in professional development and continuous improvement; it is a core aspect of career development of the professional and a requirement to institutional membership and a key constituent of lifelong learning. Modern businesses recognise the clear benefits in having professionally qualified career-minded staff and often provide mentoring and training programmes in support. Approaches to CPD activities are varied, and no one method suites all; it is better for those people attending CPD sessions not to limit attendance to one approach as different approaches can be just as useful as the event topic when learning new skills. Further, not all CPD activities have tangible CPD hours, a metric that is required as evidence to support continuing membership by Royal and Chartered institutions. This should not put of those willing to learn and improve competencies such as teamworking, which can be harder to evidence. Critical thinking can be difficult to learn, but having such skills will help the individual in both their decision-making abilities when choosing appropriate CPD activities and achieving their short- and long-term career goals.

References

Balfour Beatty. www.balfourbeatty.com
Chartered Institute of Personnel Development. www.CIPD.co.uk
Royal Institution of Chartered Surveyors. www.rics.org

2 The construction industry and CPD

2.1 Introduction

This chapter introduces the construction industry. Its size, reach, and importance are emphasised, as well as its essential nature to the very fabric of the UK (and world). The main government reports and targets, both contemporary and those historic that are still applicable, are also introduced and discussed. They include Construction 2025, The Farmer Review: Modernise or Die, and the Government's Construction Sector Deal. The Construction Leadership Council's (CLC) Future Skills Report is also discussed. All construction industry reports and professional bodies prioritise the development of construction industry professionals and reaffirm the importance of this for the future of the industry. The current and anticipated skills gap is also discussed. Ultimately, with proactive and effective Continuous Professional Development Plans staff can ensure they remain relevant in a changing professional environment and take a leadership role in their own development. This will not only improve their skill sets and career progression opportunities, but will also help contribute to a more productive construction industry.

2.2 The construction industry

The construction industry can be described as the design, development, construction, maintenance, demolition, and protection of the built and natural environment. This extends to infrastructure, engineering, and construction works; can be public or privately funded; and can span many different forms, project types, and sectors, including commercial, retail, educational, residential, healthcare, and defence. In the most recent 'Construction Industry: Statistics and Policy' briefing paper, published by the House of Commons Library at the end of 2019 and freely available online, a key overview of the UK construction industry is provided. For the past 30 years, as a percentage of the UK economy the construction industry has been between 5.1% and 6.7% (Rhodes, 2019). In 2018 the UK construction industry made up 6% of the economy and contributed some £117 billion (or up to 10% of the economy according to the CLC (2019). It is reported that construction is responsible for over 2.4 million UK jobs (6.6% of the UK total) and over 343,000 companies (13%) of UK businesses. These figures only represent companies that operate above the current value added tax (VAT) threshold of £85,000 and so there are many more companies operating in the construction industry that do not reach this threshold (Rhodes, 2016).

The number of those employed by companies operating in the construction industry is fairly static per region, with the North East the lowest region where 5.6% of jobs belong to the construction industry. This increases to 7.5% in the South West and, along with all other regions, averages to 6.6% of total UK employment. The industry is made up of primarily UK nationals, with on average 10% of the workforce classed as non-UK national (approximately three quarters of these are from within the EU). As a percentage of all jobs in UK construction nearly 37% of those are classed as self-employed, with it reported that approximately 74% of UK construction work was in the private sector with the remaining 26% public sector work (Rhodes, 2016).

In addition to over 343,000 companies operating within the construction industry, there are also professional bodies operating on behalf of trades, sectors, operatives, and professionals within the industry. Examples include the Construction Industry Council (CIC), the CLC, the Construction Industry Training Board (CITB), and the Federation of Master Builders (FMB), the Chartered Institute of Builders, the Royal Institution of Chartered Surveyors, the Institution of Civil Engineers, the Royal Institute of British Architects, and the Association for Project Managers to name a few. Many of the professional bodies are discussed throughout this book in relation to CPD, but a few are introduced below to illustrate the range of professional bodies that exist and how they all aim to improve the construction industry in their own way.

2.2.1 *The Construction Industry Training Board*

Operating across England, Scotland and Wales, the CITB aims to support the industry by attracting new talent and developing existing talent by ensuring employers have access to the training they want when they need it. The CITB is a non-departmental public body originally set up in 1964. Looking towards the future, the CITB has set out an agenda for change which includes being responsive and reforming its grant scheme; being innovative, influential, and accountable; representing the industry more effectively; and modernising to become more relevant in how they help support, develop, and improve the UK construction industry.

2.2.2 *The Construction Industry Council*

The Construction Industry Council (CIC) is a forum that represents professional bodies, specialist business associations, and research organisations in the UK construction industry. Founded in 1988 the CIC attempts to provide a single voice for built environment professionals. This voice serves to represent over 25,000 construction consultant firms and over 500,000 individual professionals. The vision of the CIC is to be respected and recognised by both the UK construction industry and government as an effective thought leader representing the UK built environment professionals (CIC 2020).

2.2.3 The Federation of Master Builders

To protect the interests of small- and medium-sized construction companies, the FMB was established in 1941 as an independent non-profit group to lobby for members interests. The FMB supports its members to become the best in the construction industry, and by offering a range of support and training, the FMB champions continuous development and improvement (FMB, 2020).

2.2.4 Many voices, one purpose

The professional bodies introduced above, as well as all those who seek to serve the construction industry, all arguably have the same ultimate purpose: to improve the construction industry. Many professional bodies represent groups, companies or professionals operating within the industry, and some even overlap in the members they serve. This could potentially cause confusion if many bodies proclaim to speak on behalf of the industry, and then have conflicting and contradictory advice.

However, even if professional bodies do not overlap in their members they serve, sometimes confusion could still possibly occur if each professional bodies advice seeks to specifically address their own members concerns without considering the wider construction industry stakeholders. Thankfully, such situations rarely occur with professional bodies often working together to serve the majority of the construction industry. Professional bodies rarely pull in different directions even though they may be representing different members interests. This is because ultimately the all professional bodies are aware of what makes a successful construction industry: professionals pulling together, working collaboratively, and continuously improving their skills.

However, despite the availability of such leadership, and the unanimous support of all professional bodies for the continuous professional development of their members, and the shared aim of improving the construction industry, the industry has historically been slow to adopt new practices and has suffered from what has been described as a productivity problem.

2.3 A construction industry productivity problem

The Office for National Statistics (ONS) is an institute recognised for its wide-ranging national data sets and is the UK's largest independent producer of statistics. It reports directly to the UK Parliament but is a non-ministerial department. The main responsibility of the ONS is to collect, analyse, and disseminate statistics regarding the UK's economy, society, and population. Data is published in over 600 releases each year, and further statistical information can also be requested on an individual or institutional basis. The ONS also runs an annual Research Excellence Award which aims to recognise and celebrate outstanding innovative research conducted using the data it produces that delivers public benefits.

For the economy as a whole, as well as its constituent industries, output per hour expressed in pounds is often the measure of productivity. The ONS produces all relevant and applicable productivity information and its data reveals many interesting findings. First, data from the ONS reveals that the average productivity of the whole economy has only marginally improved between the period of Q1 2007 and Q4 2017 from 32.5 to 33.7. In the same time period, the construction industry has improved from 24.0 to 27.0 (ONS, 2018). However, this is still far below the average of the UK economy. Such figures look especially worrying when you consider the services sector, manufacturing, production and agriculture, and the finance sector; all outperformed the construction industry across the same time period. Financial services are by far the most economically productive but have actually decreased from 2007 to 2017 from 68.9 to 66.4.

There have been many commentators who have considered the 'productivity problem' afflicting the UK construction industry from many different angles; to date, nothing appears to be successfully reversing the trend. However, there are some initiatives and reports that offer possible solutions, and the future of the construction industry from this point forward could be disrupted through innovative approaches and technologies. If the industry resists such innovation and fails to embrace potential technology, then according to the Farmer Review, the construction industry as we know it will die. In part to help address this productivity problem, and to help prepare the industry for the future, the UK government released its strategy entitled 'Construction 2025'.

2.4 Construction 2025

Construction 2025 is an industrial strategy launched by the UK government in July 2013. It outlines the government's long-term vision of how the government and construction industry will work together "*to put Britain at the forefront of global construction...*" (HM Government, 2013). The strategy sets ambitious targets for the industry such as lowering initial construction costs and whole life cycle by 33%, reducing the time taken from inception to completion of projects by 50%, lowering greenhouse gas emissions by 50%, and reducing the total trade gap between exports and imports by 50% for construction materials products. Construction 2025 also sets out what it wants to achieve by highlighting its clear vision with five aims. These are discussed in the sections that follow.

2.4.1 People – an industry that is known for its talented and diverse workforce

Whilst the industry already has some great people working within it, the overall number of staff needed in the construction sector is forecast to increase, and the skills needed to both thrive as an individual and thrive as a whole industry need to be developed. One of the first intentions of this strategy is to promote the industry as an ideal place to work and inspire the younger generations to move into the sector for employment, making it an industry of choice. The strategy wants a coordinated approach by all stakeholders and increased engagement with bodies across the industry to improve the image of construction. However, in addition to improving the image to encourage greater recruitment, the strategy also presses for the workforce to be capable and highly trained in order to truly transform the industry over the coming decades.

The Government sees the benefit of continuous professional development for construction sector professionals, and the need for CPD to ensure all workers remain agile and ready to both meet the future demands of the industry and lead the industry itself into the future.

2.4.2 *Smart – an industry that is efficient and technologically advanced*

Building upon the UK's world-class science and research base, this strategy aims to exploit developed innovative solutions for the good of the industry to help achieve all targets set. The strategy calls for investment in smart construction and digital design, bringing forward all research and innovation and for the widespread adoption of Building Information Modelling (BIM). Construction 2025 calls for the fulfilment of the Digital Built Britain Agenda and a more interlinked and closer working relationship between the industry and academic and research communities.

2.4.3 *Sustainable – an industry that leads the world in low-carbon and green construction exports*

Wider environmental considerations is called for in everything that is built, from how and why we build to the energy performance of what we build to meet the increase in demand for green and sustainable projects. Procurement of construction works is major focus to help achieve this aim. This strategy looks at all clients, public and private, to take responsibility for how construction projects are procured and to focus on reducing waste throughout the supply chain, allocating risk effectively and promoting innovation and wider value for money.

Low-carbon construction also needs to be embraced to take advantage of the growing green economy and increase focus upon sustainable agendas. This will inevitably open up a skills gap that needs to be addressed, with the right people developed correctly to meet this need when it arises and push the sustainable agenda forward. The reduction of carbon will be led by the Green Construction Board (part of the CLC) with the strategy also calling for the pipeline of future construction work available to be more transparent to all users and all procurement activities to be made more efficient.

2.4.4 *Growth – an industry that drives growth across the entire economy*

Globally construction will increase predominantly in emerging economies which can result in opportunities to expand its reach for the UK construction industry. With the population set to expand from 7.2 billion to 9 billion by the mid-2050s, Construction 2025 identifies democratic shifts in countries that will present major built environment and natural resource challenges that the UK will be able to positively contribute to. This strategy also focuses on the creation of a strong and robust supply chain, which is especially important in the construction industry as it is predominantly made up of small- and medium-sized enterprises. Construction 2025 wants access to funding increased for all the supply chain, and also an improvement in the payment practices they face. Lastly, the strategy wants the industry to identify and take advantage of any global opportunities that are presented due to the increasing worldwide need and demand.

2.4.5 Leadership – an industry with clear leadership from a CLC

Construction 2025 stands firmly behind the CLC and backs it to provide the leadership and guidance the industry needs to meet the demands of the future. This strategy's vision for 2025 (which is fast approaching) is outlined over five points that are listed below:

1 An industry that attracts and retains a diverse group of multi-talented people, operating under considerably safer and healthier conditions, which has become a sector of choice for young people inspiring them into rewarding professional and vocational careers
2 A UK industry that leads the world in research and innovation, transformed by digital design, advanced materials, and new technologies, fully embracing the transition to a digital economy and the rise of smart construction
3 An industry that has become dramatically more sustainable through its efficient approach to delivering low-carbon assets more quickly and at a lower cost, underpinned by strong, integrated supply chains and productive long-term relationships
4 An industry that drives and sustains growth across the entire economy by designing, manufacturing, building, and maintaining assets which deliver genuine whole-life value for customers in expanding markets both at home and abroad
5 An industry with clear leadership from a CLC that reflects a strong and enduring partnership between industry and government

Construction 2025 goes further and conducts a SWOT on the construction industry (SWOTs are explored in more detail in Chapter 4). These include Strengths such as the wider economic significance of the industry, its large supply chain, and world-class design skills. The Weaknesses of the industry include low-sector integration, low levels of innovation, and a lack of knowledge sharing and collaboration. This strategy also identifies Opportunities the construction industry can take advantage of such as implementing BIM, growing in emerging markets, and the ability to adopting low-carbon construction methods. Finally, the Threats to the construction industry are highlighted, and these include access to finance for SMEs, low training and skills shortages, and a high degree of fragmentation.

Describing the current situation in the UK construction industry, Construction 2025 states that

> despite high redundancy and low vacancy rates, the industry continues to face significant skills shortages, with almost one fifth of all vacancies classified as hard to fill. These shortages are evident mainly in skilled trades and professional occupations. This leads to inefficiency in the way the industry operates and reduces its overall competitiveness.
>
> (HM Government, 2013, p. 44)

In summary, Construction 2025 is a call to arms for the industry to improve in order to survive and thrive in the future. It identifies the current failings of the industry and discusses how these failings can be addressed by all members of the supply chain. If the points of the strategy are dissected at a more granular and actionable level, it becomes clear that organisations operating within the construction industry need to invest in the training and development of their staff – ultimately therefore, if the construction industry is to meet any of the targets set to thrive in the future, the professionals who operate within it need to develop their skill sets.

2.5 Construction Leadership Council

The CLC were initially tasked by the UK government to look at the labour model in the construction industry, and it was the CLC that in turn commissioned Mark Farmer.

Established in 2013 the CLC oversees the implementation of government construction strategies. The CLC works between the government and the construction industry to identify and deliver actions that will support UK construction to build greater efficiency, growth, and skills – mainly the objective of the CLC is to drive industry improvement and achieve the targets set out in the government's construction 2025 strategy and to drive the industry towards smarter construction. The CLC define smart construction as follows:

> Smart Construction is the design, construction and operation of assets achieved through collaborative partnerships which make full use of digital technologies and industrialised manufacturing techniques to improve productivity, minimise whole life costs, improve sustainability and maximise user benefits.
>
> (CLC, 2018)

The CLC (2020a) themselves state that their main focus is upon:

- Digital – delivering better, more certain outcomes by using BIM-enabled ways of working
- Manufacturing – increasing the proportion of off-site manufacture to improve productivity, quality, and safety
- Whole-life performance – getting more out of new and existing assets through the use of smart technologies.

There are six work streams the CLC uses to identify and explore how the desired outcomes can be delivered; these include the following:

- Supply Chain and Business
- Smart Technology
- Exports and Trades
- Skills
- Innovation in Buildings
- Green Construction

Whilst all of the six CLC work streams are important to a modern and thriving construction industry, the one that is directly applicable to the development of construction industry professionals is 'skills'. This work stream focuses upon developing a skilled UK construction workforce. According to the CLC,

> It is critical that the workforce of today and tomorrow have the right skills to meet the needs of the construction industry and are able to deliver our ambitions of a more efficient, productive, lower carbon, more innovative construction industry. The work stream will focus on creating a shared and sustainable framework which delivers a workforce with the relevant skills to match the industry's needs.
>
> (CLC, 2020b)

The CLC go on to say that for the construction industry to thrive it needs to retain and recruit talented professionals who have the right skill sets – and these skill sets then need to be continuously updated with the evolving nature and demands of the construction industry. This adds weight to the argument of continuous professional development and therefore should form part of any future discussion under this work stream by the CLC.

In June 2019 the CLC published their 'Future Skills Report' (CLC, 2019). In the report the CLC highlight the changing nature of the construction industry and discuss the need to both anticipate the future skills professionals will require, and also a need to focus on the skills crisis that currently exists. The report goes further and says the skills required for the future of construction work fall into one of the following four categories:

a Digital skills – to enable and improve productivity, clear digital leadership is required throughout the industry
b Technical skills – aimed at smart construction methods at all stages of a project life cycle, allowing smart solutions to be designed and manufactured at an early stage rather than only being considered towards the end of the project delivery
c Collaborative skills – to assist effective teamwork as projects become more complex, demanding, and interconnected.
d Traditional skills – the maintenance and enhancement of traditional skills is also imperative to avoid skills shortages.

The report goes on to argue that it is fear of not seeing a return on investment in training that is holding the construction industry back from embracing the costs and time associated with long-term staff development. However, the Future Skills Report does put forward three headline actions that will have a positive impact on the skills of construction industry staff; these are as follows:

1 Clients to agree a code of employment where all those individuals involved in the delivery of a project are directly employed, thereby ensuring it is in an employer's best interests to train their staff as this will assist their own productivity.

2 An environment needs to flourish where smart construction methods are encouraged at early stages of a project. This will create a demand for skilled employees which then drives employers to invest in staff.
3 Applicable industry qualifications and training is updated to include smart construction techniques and behaviours and more funding to train is made available.

Whilst the encouragement of the construction industry to enhance the skills of its workforce is admirable, and the CLC outline the many benefits of this and methods the government and clients can use to encourage the rest of the industry to take note, the overwhelming message is that the construction industry is evolving. Whilst traditional skill sets will still be needed for the foreseeable future, there is a real need for a more enhanced set of skills to meet both the immediate and future requirements of the construction industry. Ultimately therefore, if companies across the industry are not investing in their employees, such employees should arguably take responsibility for their own development. Whist this will inevitably be more difficult without all companies' support, encouragement, and financial backing, it appears that the companies that don't encourage staff development won't be ready to meet the future demands of the construction industry. Therefore, there is a good chance that those companies won't be around to experience the future of construction. As an individual, if you have the right skill sets, you will inevitably find it easier to find employment and to move more easily to companies that thrive because they invest in the training and development of staff, or, as Mark Farmer puts it, companies will have to "*modernise or die*".

2.6 The Farmer Review

The Farmer Review of the UK Construction Labour Model: Modernise or Die – Time to Decide the Industry's Future (or Farmer Review for short) is a British government commissioned construction industry report. It was published by the CLC in 2016 and was led by Mark Farmer.

Mark Farmer has over 30 years' experience in the construction industry and is a Founding Director and CEO of a construction industry consultancy called 'Cast'. Cast is a specialist consultancy focusing on the UK residential development and investment market. Cast derives its name from a community of Harris's Hawks, and it aims to embrace innovation, technology, and the Design for Manufacture agenda to help improve productivity, performance, and predictability in the construction industry.

The Farmer Review adopts a medical analogy in its undertaking and presenting of construction industry research and follows the process of identifying any symptoms, diagnosing the root causes, providing a prognosis, establishing a treatment plan for recovery, and finally keeping the industry under observation. The many 'symptoms' of the construction industry are immediately identified as low predictability, structural fragmentation, leadership fragmentation, low margins, adversarial pricing models and financial fragility, a dysfunctional training and delivery model, workforce size and demographics, lack of collaboration and improvement culture, lack of research and development in innovation, and a poor public

Table 2.1 The authors summary of the Farmer Review recommendations and UK Government responses

	Farmer Review recommendation	*UK Government response*
1	The CLC should be responsible for implementing the recommendations set out in the Farmer Review.	The Government agrees but says it is for the CLC to decide and is setting an example themselves of better collaboration in procurement and through the use of BIM.
2	The CITB should be reformed.	The CITB should be retained but reformed. This is currently being undertaken by the CITB and supported by the Government.
3	Industry, clients, and Government should collaborate more to improve relationships and invest in research and development within the industry.	The CLC should continue to develop better models of client commissioning, focusing on collaboration.
4	Industry, clients, Government, and academia should work together to invest in and implement innovation across the industry.	The Government will drive BIM through procurement practices and allow access to funding to support innovation.
5	A reformed CITB should consider how its grant funding can promote skills and training to meet the future demands of the industry.	The Government agrees with the CLC encouraged to take a leadership role in pushing the industry forward towards modernisation.
6	A reformed CITB should have more responsibility and engage in an outreach school programme to help improve the industry's image and vision for the future.	The Government reaffirmed its commitment to increasing apprentice and degree apprentice numbers and agrees the industry needs to present a positive image.
7	The Government should recognise the importance of the construction industry and help maintain the required skills capacity.	The Government has published a Green Paper on its industrial strategy and has introduced a sector deal.
8	The Government should promote innovation in the housing sector by promoting the use of pre-manufactured solutions.	The Government has announced over £25 billion of investment to increase housing supply.
9	A comprehensive pipeline of demand should be published by the Government.	A National Infrastructure and Construction Pipeline was published in December 2016.
10	The Government should consider an additional charge on construction clients to drive change if they do not adopt it on their own.	The Government agrees the involvement of clients is crucial; however, client charges won't be introduced as they may damage client confidence and increase costs.

imagine. Low productivity is also highlighted as one of the main symptoms of the current construction industry. The findings of the Review reinforce the points made earlier in this book regarding the poor productivity of the construction industry. The Review also goes wider and states that the problem of low productivity in the construction industry is not just limited to the UK, but that the US and other international markets have also suffered from the same issues (Farmer, 2016).

In the diagnosis of the symptoms, three root causes are identified: the industry adopting a survivalist mentality, non-aligned client and industry interests, and no strategic incentive to initiative transformational change. The report also discusses how the industry could witness a 25% decline in the availability of its workforce within the next ten years undermining the ability of the UK construction industry to deliver the core construction, infrastructure, and engineering projects required. The report's prognosis is that if the construction industry does not take immediate action at this critical crossroads, then the risks could become overwhelming and the industry could become debilitated. The recommended plan for action is based around a requirement for strong leadership throughout the industry, particularly for governments to drive change through regulation and clients to take responsibility for leading the industry through a period of change via their commissioning behaviours.

The Farmer Review cumulates in ten headline recommendations. On the 19th May 2017, the UK government formally responded to the Farmer Review. The formal response includes individual responses to each of the ten recommendations set out in the Review (HM Government, 2017). The recommendations from the Farmer Review and the government responses are set out in Table 2.1.

Whilst the Farmer Review does comprehensively consider many aspects of the wider construction industry in its remit, the problems it identifies ultimately come down to a lack of clear communication, leadership, and direction for the future. A common denominator that underpins these requirements is the development of construction industry professionals. Better developed and skilled professionals are ultimately required to facilitate the leadership the construction industry needs to ensure it meets future challenges successfully.

2.7 Building a safer future

'Building a Safer Future: Independent Review of Building Regulations and Fire Safety' was published in May 2018 by Dame Judith Hackitt. The review was announced in the wake of the Grenfell Tower disaster and focused on high-rise residential buildings. However, as part of this review Dame Hackitt touched upon the skills development of construction industry professionals (Hackitt, 2018).

Whilst the connection between a report on fire safety and professional development may not appear immediately explicit, Dame Hackitt was somewhat critical of current CPD standards and practices undertaken throughout the construction industry and dedicated an entire chapter of the report to competence. The report establishes how there is "*a lack of skills, knowledge and experience...*" amongst professionals and sets out a series of recommendations to help prevent a repeat of the Grenfell Tower disaster and also increase the general competence of all construction professionals.

One of the report's recommendations is that construction leadership should capture key lessons learnt from both within and outside of the construction industry, and these lessons should then form part of staff development in an effort to increase competence levels. The report also argues that development should be meaningful with the completion of continuous development mandatory for professional body-accredited staff. The report also calls for a new competence framework and that competent staff should supervise and work closely with others to increase general competence levels. All companies should also engage with continuous improvement at all delivery levels, from manufacture, installation, advice, training, regulation, and testing bodies. Dame Hackitt does go on to stress that qualifications and training are only part of the solution and that CPD should be undertaken throughout a career to ensure competence levels remain high.

2.8 Centre for Digital Built Britain

The Centre for Digital Built Britain (CDBB) aims to deliver a smart digital economy for infrastructure and construction. The intention is to transform the construction industry's approach to planning, building, maintaining, and using the social and economic infrastructure. The CDBB itself is a partnership between the University of Cambridge and the Department for Business, Energy and Industrial Strategy.

> Digital Built Britain seeks to digitise the entire life-cycle of our built assets finding innovative ways of delivering more capacity out of our existing social and economic infrastructure, dramatically improving the way these assets deliver social services to deliver improved capacity and better public services.
>
> (University of Cambridge, 2020)

The CDBB has seven core objectives, including to act as the national and international custodian of the UK built Britain programmes, support the industry adoption of BIM, and liaise with bodies to create and modify technical standards, and ensuring that Digital Built Britain is aligned with new academic developments. The objectives also include assisting the UK to successfully exploit new technological developments, inspiring the construction industry to adopt new digital approaches, and the co-ordination and delivery of events and activities to engage the industry and to share findings to influence future policy and practice.

Whilst BIM is central to the digital transformation targets for the built environment, it can be argued that the wider remit of the CDBB is to ensure construction industry stakeholders have the knowledge and skill sets required to push the digital agenda forward and utilise both the current and future digital tools available to companies and individuals. Therefore, the CDBB could be considered to be concerned with the professional development of construction industry professionals. As it is only by developing the skill sets of current and future professionals that the Digital Built Britain agenda will be achieved.

2.9 The future of the construction industry

The construction industry is, however, not as adverse to change and development as is often reported. The Green Construction Board (GCB) set up in 2011 is part of the CLC and is an example of how the industry is seeking to address environmental concerns and sustainable leadership. The GCB has set out guidance documents on topics such as the circular economy, low-carbon constriction methods, and water management planning. There has also been a recent drive behind modern methods of construction (MMC). This is a wide term that embraces a range of house-building techniques relating to the off-site manufacture and on-site installation of houses. Several examples of current best practices and the impact such practices are having on the industry can be found in the 'Modern methods of construction; Who's doing what?' publication released by the National House Building Council (NHBC) in 2018.

However, according to the World Economic Forum (WEF) report 'Shaping the Future of Construction: A Breakthrough in Mindset and Technology' released in May 2016, a reduction in greenhouse gas emissions is one area the construction industry of the future will have to address. The UK government has set a target to reduce the 2016 levels of greenhouse gas emissions of the construction industry by 50% by 2025 as globally 30% of greenhouse gas emissions are attributable to buildings. Worldwide the construction industry is also faced with a housing crisis, increased scrutiny from all stakeholders, a skills shortage and knowledge gap, and uncertain political decision-making. The same WEF report also outlines population increase as a major factor the construction industry has to deal with as it states the population of the world's urban areas are increasing by around 200,000 people per day, placing demands on housing, transport infrastructure, and utilities. Society is also faced with an ageing population, ageing infrastructure, scarcity of resources, an increase in the frequency of 'natural' disasters, higher demand placed on food production, rising water levels, and an increased risk of global pandemics. In an attempt to tackle such problems and achieve any of the government targets set, the WEF report outlines an industry transformation framework consisting of future best practices across a variety of disciplines and levels. This includes government-level best practices covering regulation and policies, and public procurement; sector-level best practices such as industry collaboration and joint industry marketing; and company-level best practices. These cover technology, materials, and tools; processes and operations; strategy and business model innovation, and, perhaps most importantly, people, organisation and culture.

The WEF report acknowledges that at the heart of this best practice lies 'Continuous training and knowledge management' (WEF, 2016). The skills required to meet future challenges need to start to be developed early in the career of construction professionals so that they are ready to meet challenges in an innovative and proactive manner. CPD therefore is of the upmost importance for all construction professionals. If a construction professional only completes training when first entering the industry, and then goes on to have a career spanning 50 years, which is potentially five decades of employment with no further targeted development. It is no wonder therefore that the construction industry suffers from a productivity problem and, despite innovative advances in some areas, is largely held back by clients unwilling to take risks on new concepts and ideas if they are to be delivered by an untrained and traditionally minded workforce. It is for this reason that some companies heavily invest in the CPD of their staff and why for many professional bodies annual CPD is a mandatory requirement (explored in Chapter 3).

2.10 Conclusion

The construction industry is one of the most important contributors to the UK economy. Its size, scale, and the very nature of its business mean that it substantially impacts our entire society. However, the industry has historically suffered from a lack of productivity when compared to both other industries and the UK economic average – a problem that is still evident today. To address this productivity problem, the UK government commissions reports and reviews, releases research and development funding, supports the development of industry bodies, and encourages modern approaches to construction in its own projects. We can therefore see that the UK government has clear intentions to modernise the construction industry, and the numerous reports, bodies, and frameworks set up have the aim of helping achieve this agenda. When you explore beyond and behind the headline-grabbing statements and action plans, it is revealed that all reports are largely underpinned with addressing productivity. Ultimately, this productivity is addressed by the development of construction professionals. This is a message that is echoed by all professional bodies, construction industry reviews and reports. All key stakeholders share the ultimate aim of increasing and improving the continuing professional development of construction professionals.

All professionals need to ensure their skill sets are not only up to date with current best practices but proactively prepared to meet the challenges of the future. Some companies are starting to realise that encouraging staff development and empowerment results in a productive and powerful workforce of professionals. If the Farmer Review is correct in its worst-case forecasts in that those companies that do not modernise and fail to become more productive will ultimately die, it will be those companies that do embrace technology, look to the future, and develop their workforce that will survive. That is not to say everyone should leave their current companies if they are not developing you at this particular time, although it may be a factor in leading you to look for employment elsewhere, for a company that does support your development needs. However, it is always worth

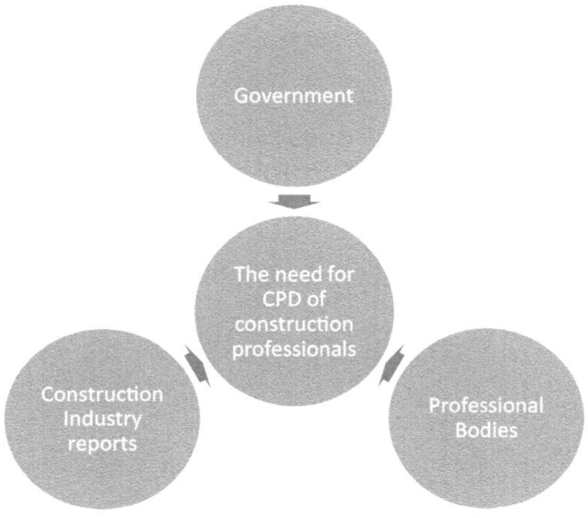

Figure 2.1 The Construction Industry and CPD

being conscious of your own development and remembering that even if the current company you are employed by doesn't develop its staff as long you you take responsibility for your own development you will be in a much stronger position when your current company that does not invest in its workforce inevitably fails.

References

Construction Industry Council (2020). *Construction Industry Council*. Available from: http://cic.org.uk/about-us/

Construction Leadership Council (2018). *Smart Construction. A Guide for Housing Clients*. Available from: https://www.constructionleadershipcouncil.co.uk/wp-content/uploads/2018/10/181010-CLC-Smart-Construction-Guide.pdf

Construction Leadership Council (2019). *Future Skills Report*. Accessed from: http://www.constructionleadershipcouncil.co.uk/wp-content/uploads/2019/06/CLC-Skills-Workstream_Future-Skills-Report_June-2019_A4-Print-Version.pdf

Construction Leadership Council (2020a). *The Construction Leadership Council*. Accessed from: http://www.constructionleadershipcouncil.co.uk/about/

Construction Leadership Council (2020b). *Skills Work Stream*. Accessed from: http://www.constructionleadershipcouncil.co.uk/workstream/skills/

Farmer, M (2016). *The Farmer Review of the UK Construction Labour Model. Modernise or Die. Time to Decide the Industry's Future*. Construction Leadership Council. Available from: https://www.constructionleadershipcouncil.co.uk/wp-content/uploads/2016/10/Farmer-Review.pdf

Federation of Master Builders (2020). *About the FMB*. Available from: https://www.fmb.org.uk/about-the-fmb/

Hackitt, J. (2018). *Building a Safer Future. Independent Review of Building Regulations and Fire Safety*. Final Report. Available from: https://assets.publishing.service.gov.uk/government/uploads/system/uploads/attachment_data/file/707785/Building_a_Safer_Future_-_web.pdf

HM Government (2013). *Industrial Strategy: Government and Industry in Partnership, Construction 2025*. Available from: https://assets.publishing.service.gov.uk/government/uploads/system/uploads/attachment_data/file/210099/bis-13-955-construction-2025-industrial-strategy.pdf

HM Government (2017). *Modernise or Die: The Farmer Review of the UK Construction Labour Model*. Government Response. Available from: https://assets.publishing.service.gov.uk/government/uploads/system/uploads/attachment_data/file/630457/farmer-review-construction-labour-model-government-response.pdf

NHBC Foundation (2018). *Modern Methods of Construction. Who's Doing What?*. Available from: https://www.nhbcfoundation.org/wp-content/uploads/2018/11/NF82.pdf

Office of National Statistics (2018). *Construction Statistics, Great Britain: 2017*. Available at: https://www.ons.gov.uk/businessindustryandtrade/constructionindustry/articles/constructionstatistics/number192018edition#comparisons-and-contributions-to-the-economy

Rhodes, C. (2016). *Construction Industry: Statistics and Policy*. Nr 01432. House of Commons Library.

Rhodes, C. (2019). *Construction Industry: Statistics and Policy*. Nr 01432. House of Commons Library.

University of Cambridge (2020). *Centre for Digital Built Britain*. Available from: https://www.cdbb.cam.ac.uk/AboutCDBB

World Economic Forum (2016). *Shaping the Future of Construction. A Breakthrough in Mindset and Technology*. Available from: http://www3.weforum.org/docs/WEF_Shaping_the_Future_of_Construction_full_report__.pdf

3 Professional bodies in the construction industry

3.1 Introduction

This chapter discusses, in the authors views, the role of different professional bodies. Those that operate mainly in the construction industry are discussed such as the Royal Institution of Chartered Surveyors (RICS), the Chartered Institute of Building (CIOB), the Association for Project Management (APM), the Institution of Civil Engineers (ICE), and the Royal Institute of British Architects (RIBA). Professional bodies that are also relevant to the industry are discussed, such as the Chartered Institute of Procurement and Supply (CIPS), and the Institute of Chartered Accountants England and Wales (ICAEW). Each professional body is introduced, with membership levels and obligations for entry explored. The continuing professional development (CPD) requirements of each professional body are then considered as are the professional body rules and regulations. How such requirements can be achieved and any applicable rules and regulations can be abided by are also discussed. Finally this chapter cumulates in an analysis of professional body CPD requirements and a comparison highlighting the similarities in all professional body requirements, expectations, and importance when it comes to professional development. In order to achieve and maintain the membership of any professional body, as well as improving your skills and competency levels whilst staying up to date with contemporary industry development, CPD is a concept that must be engaged with by organisations and individuals alike. This chapter reveals the consistent importance the role of CPD has amongst leading industry bodies and therefore reveals the importance with which all construction industry professionals should treat CPD.

3.2 What is a professional body?

A professional body is an organisation that usually sits within a single profession or industry that consists of individual members who aim to promote best practices and set the standards and expectations of behaviour for both members and the wider profession. This is often executed by the introduction of codes of conduct and by requiring all members to undertake formal and informal professional development each year. Professional bodies also often strive to do more, and to be more. For example, charitable arms of professional bodies have been established for the benefit of both wider society and the professional body members themselves who fall upon hard times. Professional bodies also often go above and beyond the setting of standards for their own members and try to influence the behaviour of the wider industries in which they operate through the release of free-to-use educational handbooks and guides. Often professional bodies also find themselves as the representatives of an industry and release statements or contribute to news segments when an industrial and expert opinion is sought. At its core, a professional body is a group of likeminded individuals operating to improve the standards of their profession and are willing to and often elected to speak on its behalf.

When one or more professional bodies exist within the profession or industry, there can be a large amount of crossover, as they will inevitably be commenting on the same issues. Whilst this is not uncommon, it is rare for the professional bodies to disagree. Each body will have its own approach, and often its own unique publications and distinctive voice – but ultimately its aims will be the same. There are also differences between professional bodies operating within the same sphere, whether these are abundantly obvious or more nuanced, each body will offer something unique to its members and will rarely prevent members from seeking simultaneous membership of another professional body. Where differences do appear in formal communications from professional bodies operating with an overlap, this will be from a different perspective of focus, and rarely from clashes over what is and isn't appropriate and applicable to the industry or profession(s) in question.

The existence of professional bodies has largely revolved around the CPD of its members and promoting best practices and ethical standards, with their intentions to promote the best aspects and eliminate the worst aspects of a particular profession or industry. Ethics often go above and beyond what is legally required and provide a framework of desired behaviours against which we hold ourselves accountable. For example, it may not be illegal to take credit for a colleague's work behind their back, but many would certainly consider such behaviour unethical – and such behaviour would definitely fall foul of professional body's expected behavioural standards. Ethics is also an issue that brings many professional bodies together. For example, the International Ethics Standards Coalition aims to create a universal set of ethical principles in the real estate and construction industries. The coalition first met in 2014 and released its International Ethics Standards in 2016 (IES-C, 2016). The IESC is made up of over 100 professional bodies from around the world and is a great example of different professional bodies sharing resources and working collaboratively to develop an international standard that they can all adopt.

Some bodies allow members to voluntarily sign up with little or no oversight; others have stringent entry requirements and award membership to candidates who pass these successfully. Sometimes a rigorous review of a potential applicants' professional experience is conducted, whilst for some professional bodies membership can be automatic, or with less scrutiny, if you fulfil stipulated criteria, for example if a candidate has over a certain amount of years of managerial experience and is the member of a separate respected professional body. Once an individual is a member of a professional body, there are often levels of membership that can be ascended. The number of levels available is dependent upon the professional body itself, but memberships can include grades such as student or junior member, trainee, member, fellow, and senior fellow to name just a few. Membership grade could also be identified by a numbered ranking system, with lower numbers the entry positions of membership and higher numbers achieved and awarded for experience and responsibility and the successful completion of set requirements.

3.3 Professional bodies in the construction industry

There are many professional bodies operating within the construction industry and many more that cover professionals both inside and outside of the industry. They all ultimately have the same purpose and similar aims, but specific to their own members. Often professional bodies will also work in conjunction with one another to add emphasis to any joint publications and show unity when it comes to important issues that transcend single professions and industrial sectors. Some of the professional bodies that are important to the construction industry are explored in more detail with their specific entry requirements and levels of membership discussed.

3.3.1 Royal Institution of Chartered Surveyors

The RICS can trace its history back to 1792 with the formation of the Surveyors Club. From this the 'Institute of Surveyors' was then founded in London in 1868, and the professional body received its Royal Charter in 1881, before becoming officially known as the Royal Institution of Chartered Surveyors in 1947. Operating on behalf of valuation, management, and development of land, real estate, construction, and infrastructure professionals, the RICS states that it "*delivers confidence through respected global standards, adopted and enforced by over 134,000 qualified and trainee professionals across the built and natural environment*" (RICS, 2020a).

There are different levels of membership at the RICS and different progression routes once you are a member. However, the membership levels are the same regardless of profession – all members will be classed from the same range of designation. Table 3.1 provides a brief overview of the RICS membership options.

In order to be eligible to join the RICS as either an Associate Member or a Chartered Member, an individual will have had to complete a minimum of 48 hours' CPD per 12 months they have been registered on the RICS membership process. This process for the Chartered Member route to entry is called the Assessment of Professional Competence (APC). If you have ten or more years of experience in your profession, you can progress straight to the final assessment following a preliminary review of your submitted documents. If, however, you do not have ten or more years of experience, you will undertake a period of structured

Table 3.1 An overview of RICS membership options

Levels of membership	*The authors view on the levels of membership*
Associate Member (AssocRICS)	Membership is gained by completing the associate qualification once you have met the required entry requirements. These range from one year's experience with a degree to four years' minimum experience without any qualifications. The assessment process takes between 6 and 12 months to complete, with individuals needing to complete an online ethics course, summarise their experience in 3,000 words, and write a 2,500-word case study report on a project they have been involved in. A record of at least 48 hours of CPD in the preceding 12 months will also need to be provided.
Chartered Member (MRICS)	Membership is gained by completing the chartered qualification and can be applied for once a candidate has amassed the relevant experience and achieved a RICS-accredited degree. You can also apply for this level with five years' experience with any degree or at least ten years' experience operating at a senior level. The most common process of entry is through the APC (discussed later in this chapter).
RICS Fellow (FRICS)	This membership grade is a mark of distinction and demonstrates a high level of professional achievement. In order to achieve this, you will first have to be MRICS qualified, and then illustrate you have acted to further the RICS and your profession, reflected the RICS' public interest mandate, and promoted the RICS' objectives.

training and development for either 12 or 24 months before submission of your final documents for review. Twelve months of structured training is required if you have more than five years of experience with twenty-four months of structured training required for anyone with less than five years of experience. If the review is successful, you will then be invited to a final interview where your submitted documents, training plan, CPD record, and wider industry and RICS knowledge will be assessed. This will be against three levels of attainment:

- Level 1 – Knowledge and understanding
- Level 2 – Application of knowledge and understanding
- Level 3 – Reasoned advice and depth of knowledge.

The APC itself is a structured process whereby a candidate must keep a record of their development against a set of competencies that consist of both general competencies applicable to all RICS members and specific competencies to the individual's professional sector. As part of the RICS the candidate will appoint a supervisor and councillor to help support their journey and have to complete all requirements before submitting their documents. The 12- and 24-month time frames are the minimum with many candidates taking longer.

3.3.1.1 CPD requirements for the RICS

One common requirement for all candidates is the need to keep CPD records. For those aspiring to be Associate Members and Chartered Members, 48 hours of CPD must be recorded each year of the training. The RICS views CPD as a "*commitment by members to continually update their skills and knowledge in order to remain professionally competent*" (RICS, 2020d). This CPD must be split between formal and informal activities, with Table 3.2 illustrating the main differences.

Activities that do not have a clear learning outcome, are not structured or planned, and are not relevant to your role, profession or industry is unlikely to be applicable formal or informal CPD. To help a member understand if an activity can be counted as CPD, and if so whether it is formal or informal, the RICS has published a one-page 'CPD Decision Tree' that can be downloaded. RICS CPD requirements are also not limited to those individuals wanting to become members, but also apply to all current members across all grades of membership. Once a member of the RICS however, it is deemed that you will develop and improve your skills naturally in your day-to-day responsibilities, and so the amount of CPD hours recorded is reduced to 20 per calendar year.

Discussion 3.1

What are the advantages and disadvantages of having a set minimum annual CPD hour requirement?

The requirement to complete the 20 hours each year, 10 of which must be formal, is an important part of the RICS and key to what being a Chartered professional means. The RICS decided to set the 20-hour minimum requirement so as not to burden members disproportionately, but act as a minimum requirement the RICS, its governing body, and members believe to be acceptable. The RICS Rules

Table 3.2 Formal and informal CPD

Type of CPD	*The authors view on the types of CPD*
Formal	It is also known as structured CPD. This is where there are clear learning outcomes and CPD objectives. For example, this could include some training courses developed and delivered by a third party on a specific topic. Self-directed learning could also be applicable where clear learning outcomes have been planned and achieved that are aligned with an individual's development needs.
Informal	This largely refers to self-managed learning that is relevant to your role, profession or industry. Training courses by a colleague, or knowledge sharing meetings, events, and seminars. It will be more difficult to provide evidence for this type of CPD activity, and so detailed records will need to be kept of the reason why it was undertaken and the learning outcome that was achieved.

of Conduct for Members and the Rules of Conduct for Firms both make explicit reference to the CPD rules that members and firms, respectively, must abide by. Failure to do so can result in membership termination and RICS expulsion. The rules also apply to all future members and firms, and so individuals who apply for membership and are found to have not acted in accordance with the standards previously can also in some instances have their membership rejected.

The RICS has Rules of Conduct for both Firms and Members, and both are underpinned by the five principles of better regulation (RICS, 2020b; 2020c): proportionality, accountability, consistency, targeting, and transparency, and they are explored in relation to what they could mean to a members' CPD in Table 3.3.

At the time of writing the latest RICS Rules of Conduct for Members were updated with the release of version 7 that came into effect on the 2nd March 2020 (RICS, 2020b). There are several rules that are relevant to the professional member with regard to their CPD. The applicable rules and how they are potentially relevant to CPD are discussed in Table 3.4.

Similarly, the RICS Rules of Conduct for Firms themselves were last updated with the release of version 7 that came into effect on the 2nd March 2020. Again, there are several rules for firms that are relevant to both companies with responsibility for helping staff meet CPD requirements and for all embers operating within RICS registered firms. The applicable firm rules and how they can be relevant to CPD are discussed in Table 3.5.

To assist both individual members and firms in achieving their CPD requirements, the RICS also offers extensive CPD support – most notably in the form of a CPD foundation. This is a subscription service that none members are also able to subscribe to and offers an annual fee option for unlimited access to CPD courses, or the ability to purchase one-off courses on an ad hoc basis.

Table 3.3 CPD and better regulation adapted from the RICS principles of better regulation for members' CPD

Principles of better regulation	*The authors view of what they mean to a professionals' CPD*
Proportionality	In relation to CPD, this principle refers to ensuring the activity is appropriate for your role and training needs.
Accountability	Decisions must be justified, i.e. whether an individual decided to participate in a certain training activity or not. It is also important to remember that members are accountable for their actions, and so not having the correct training but carrying on anyway is not justifiable. Members need to ensure they are suitably trained for the required tasks.
Consistency	If you are responsible for the development and CPD of others, you must ensure that you are consistent in your actions and responses.
Targeting	Limited resources, such as a training budget, should be focused on developing the skills that are most in need of improvement and that are most relevant for your immediate requirements.
Transparency	You will need to ensure you can justify your CPD decisions and are transparent in the identification of and reflection upon your learning outcomes.

Table 3.4 CPD and rules member adapted from RICS Rules of Conduct for Members

RICS Rule of Conduct for Members	*The authors view of the relevance to CPD*
3. Ethical behaviour	This ranges from avoiding conflicts of interest such as only approving or attending CPD events that are run by friends or that result in a financial incentive for yourself (this also potentially contravenes the Bribery Act) to acting with integrity and having high ethical standards to ensure all CPD activity is recorded accurately.
4. Competence	Members need to ensure they act within their own competence and so should reflect on their own past performance and future requirements to identify areas that need to be developed.
5. Service	This rule requires members to have high standards of service and conduct work in a timely manner. It is therefore the responsibility of individual members to ensure they are fully trained in order to meet such standards.
6. **CPD**	This rule states that members must abide by all RICS CPD requirements. Therefore, it is of the upmost importance that members fully understand their responsibilities so they can ensure they successfully achieve them.
8. Information to RICS 9. Cooperation	Members will need to fully cooperate with all RICS requirements such as completing and uploading their CPD records annually before the deadline and ensuring they meet the required amount of CPD hours be recorded.

Table 3.5 CPD and company rules adapted from RICS Rules of Conduct for Firms

RICS Rule of Conduct for Firms	*The authors view of the relevance to CPD*
3. Professional behaviour	In order to ensure employees act with integrity and have the skill and foresight to avoid conflicts of interest before they occur, firms will need to ensure that all their employees complete suitable CPD.
4. Competence	In order to ensure all employees remain competent, it is imperative that firms have a focus on their organisational CPD and ensure all employees are fully trained to achieve their professional responsibilities.
6. **Training and CPD**	It is a formal rule that all firms have procedures in place to ensure employees have training opportunities and that all staff are adequately trained.
14. Information to RICS 15. Cooperation	Firms will need to fully cooperate with all RICS requirements such as ensuring members complete and upload their CPD records annually before the deadline and ensuring members meet the required amount of CPD hours.

As the RICS is a global body setting the standards for built environment professionals, its rules and procedures are to be observed closely by all professionals. We can conclude that if you a member of the RICS or planning on becoming a member, or if you simply want to follow the industry leading standards, then following the rules set by the RICS is a must. In regard to CPD, this means recording the correct number of hours as a minimum and ensuring the targets of formal and informal CPD are achieved. However, the RICS is not the only professional body operating in the built environment that has CPD requirements for its members to achieve.

3.3.2 Chartered Institute of Building

The CIOB is the "*world's largest and most influential professional body for construction management and leadership*" (CIOB, 2020). Founded as the 'Builders Society' in 1834, it became known as the Institute of Builders in 1884 with the purpose of promoting "*excellence in the construction of buildings and just and honourable practice in the conduct of business*" (CIOB, 2020). In 1965 the name changed once again to the Institute of Building before being known as the Chartered Institute of Building in 1980 once a Royal Charter was gained. As of their 2018 annual review, the CIOB had 45,341 registered members.

There are different levels of CIOB membership, and Table 3.6 provides a brief overview of these membership options.

Table 3.6 An overview of CIOB membership options

Levels of membership	*The authors view on the levels of membership*
Non-Chartered student grade	As a student member you are not classed as a Chartered Member. There is no review to be conducted, you can simply apply, and by being a student member, you gain access to numerous resources that will assist in the development of a great career.
CIOB Member (MCIOB)	As a member you can select between the descriptor of Chartered Construction Manager and Chartered Builder. Candidates will need to have a level 6 qualification or above, or membership of another selected professional body and either three or five years' professional experience dependent upon the qualification type you hold. Individuals need to join the CIOB as an applicant and then submit the documents required for the Professional Review (this is covered in more detail later in this chapter).
CIOB Fellow (FCIOB)	This membership grade is the highest offered by the CIOB and is a globally recognised mark of distinction. In order to achieve FCIOB, you will need at least five years' professional experience leading an organisation or people, and positively contribute to the industry, communities, or society. As an MCIOB you can apply to be a fellow with the submission of a 3,000-word report evidencing how you have led a project. You can also apply directly to be an FCIOB without prior membership – this consists of a 3,000-word report, attendance at an FCIOB workshop, and professional discussion where you are questioned by two assessors and one chair.

The extent of the level of exposure and qualifications a potential candidate has will determine the assessment they face to enter the CIOB. Once membership of the CIOB is successfully achieved, there are then requirements to continuously maintain your competence as a construction professional.

3.3.2.1 CPD requirements for the CIOB

The CIOB does state that CPD is essential for its members to complete, but it empowers its professional members to take full responsibility for the quality and quantity of their own development. To that end there are no prescriptive requirements such as a set amount of hours to complete each year. However, there is still the expectation that members complete CPD and keep an up-to-date record (which can be done via the CIOB website). The CIOB says that attending conferences and seminars can count towards CPD, as can the reading of applicable magazine and website articles, and researching new products and processes.

Discussion 3.2

What are the advantages and disadvantages of having no set minimum annual CPD requirements?

To ensure standards are maintained the CIOB does have a process called 'CPD monitoring'. This is where the CIOB routinely asks a selection of members to evidence their recent CPD record. You will have to complete a CPD reply slip with all the data requested and return it to the CIOB for confirmation.

The CPD of CIOB members is of the upmost importance and in the view of the authors CPD directly or indirectly permeated its way into many of the CIOB's "Rules and regulations of professional competence and conduct" (CIOB, 2018). A breakdown of how the applicable CIOB rules relate to CPD can be found in Table 3.7 to emphasise how CPD has always been at the core of being a CIOB member.

A now superseded guide from the CIOB entitled 'Professionalism and Integrity in Construction; Code of Professional Conduct and Rules' aimed at Chartered Building Consultancies was released on the 1st October 2015 and outlined the codes of professional conduct and scheme rules that companies must follow if they were to successfully achieve Chartered status. Whilst this guide has been replaced with the Rules and Regulations of Professional Competence and Conduct (effective from 2018 and utilised in table 3.7) it is included here to show the historical and longstanding importance placed upon CPD. Table 3.8 utilises this superseded guide to evidence how, in the authors view, these rules and codes helped govern our CPD behaviour.

To help members achieve their CPD needs, the CIOB has a CIOB Academy. The academy contains all its training and development materials such as upcoming courses that are aimed at individuals who can attend either in person or online or training solutions for companies to help them deliver suitable training to their employees.

Table 3.7 CIOB rules and the authors view of the relevance to CPD

CIOB Rule	*The authors view of the relevance to CPD*
Rules 5	Members will need to demonstrate their competence, and the ideal way in which to ensure you remain competent in a changing industry is to utilise CPD.
Rule 6	Having an up to date CPD plan and regularly developing the plan and activities undertaken is an effective method to ensure good practice is evidenced and current standards are achieved.
Rule 7 and 11	In order to act in the best interests of clients and ensure good customer care is achieved it is important to be aware of the latest legislation and professional requirements, as well as industry development so any advice is appropriate and timely. One method of staying abreast of industry developments is focusing on this in a CPD plan.
Rule 10	This rule directly relates to a member's CPD expectations, and underlines the essential nature with which CPD is viewed to ensure ongoing professionalism and competence.

Table 3.8 Superseded CIOB company rules, and codes of conduct and the authors view of the relevance to CPD

Superseded CIOB Codes of Professional Conduct	*The authors view of the relevance to CPD*
3: Inform its employees and members of the supply chain of the obligations of this Code, and monitor their compliance with it.	A company will need to ensure that all its staff are aware of CPD requirements, and that they will need to complete and record all CPD activity
5: Strive to ensure that all its work is in accordance with best practice and current standards and complies with all relevant statutory and contractual requirements	In order to ensure that staff remain aware of contemporary issues in the construction industry and are informed of the latest best practice standards CPD events should be undertaken.
12: All staff engaged in the administration of the construction process have achieved, or are working towards, appropriate qualifications and are undertaking an adequate regime of continuous professional development (CPD).	This code of professional conduct directly addresses the CPD requirements of an organisations staff. Abiding by this code can be achieved with the encouragement of all staff to reflect and undertake CPD and record such events.
13: Current knowledge of, and standards of practice in, health and safety considerations are given priority. 14: The CBC member shall try to be aware of all contemporary industry developments	The best method an organisation can employ to ensure all staff remain up to date with their skills and knowledge is by having regular CPD events arranged on a variety of important and contemporary topics.

3.3.3 *Association for Project Management*

The APM is the Chartered body for the project profession and so extends beyond construction as an industry. However, with almost all construction projects having a Project Manager, or one or more individuals at least fulfilling a project management function, the APM can be considered a professional body of high importance for the construction industry. The APM's Royal Charter was awarded

Table 3.9 Levels of APM membership

APM membership levels	*Description*
Student	This level of membership is available to full- and part-time students and those on apprenticeships. It is free to join and simply requires the completion of an application form and confirmation of your course of study.
Associate	If you are new to project management or interested in joining the profession, you can sign up online as an Associate Member. This gives you access to many of the APM resources and can help support career development to full member.
Full Member (**MAPM**)	Professionals with either five years' work experience or three years and a relevant qualification can apply to be a full member. You can also apply for direct entry if you hold a higher qualification. All routes to entry require an online application to be submitted, but depending on which route you choose, you may also have to submit two supporting statements and either a 1,500- or a 2,500-word report of your project experience.
Fellow (FAPM)	If you have five years' experience as an MAPM or can demonstrate experience of an equivalent level you can apply to be an FAPM. This involves submitting a report on your project experience, a personal statement, and two statements of support.

in 2017, and with more than 30,000 individual members and over 500 organisations involved with the APM's Corporate Partnership Programme, it is one of the largest professional bodies of its kind in Europe. The APM has different levels of membership which are explored in more detail in Table 3.9.

3.3.3.1 CPD requirements for the APM

The APM takes the CPD of its members seriously. It could be argued that CPD is at the heart of what it means to be an APM member. It considers CPD as a personal commitment by members to ensure their professional knowledge is up to date and places the requirement on members to undertake at least 35 hours of CPD each year which is randomly sampled. Such CPD activity must also include reflective statements on how the learning has been applied. The APM also undertook joint research with the Professional Development Consortium as part of a CPD Research Project and made the following recommendations (APM, 2020b):

- Keep up to date with regulatory changes that affect your role.
- Improve your job performance by learning new information, skills, attitudes, and behaviours.
- Expand and improve your professional capacity.

Table 3.10 The APM's Code of Conduct and CPD

APM's Code of Professional Conduct	*The authors view of the relevance to CPD*
4. Standards of Professional Conduct	Regular CPD will help ensure that knowledge of relevant legislation and standards is up to date.
5.1.c. Acting in the interests clients	One interpretation of how this code could relate to CPD includes that only when an individual is fully aware of all latest rules, regulations and industry developments can clients be fully advised, and their interests served. Not knowing about an opportunity or innovation that could be of benefit could be due to poor CPD and could therefore be avoided with proactive and high quality CPD management.
5.1.e. Ensuring professional skills are up to date	This element from the Code of Conduct governs the CPD behaviour of members and requires all members to complete CPD activities based around closing their own skill and knowledge gaps.

All APM members commit to undertaking the required 35 hours when they commence membership by signing up to the APM Code of Conduct (APM, 2020a). Elements of the APM's Code of Conduct directly and indirectly impact upon the CPD requirements with some examples explored in more detail in Table 3.10.

The 'mission' of the APM is "*inspiring communities to deliver meaningful change for societal benefit by advancing the art, science, theory and practice of project management*" (APM, 2020c). This mission in underpinned by the APM's five dimensions of professionalism that help professional development whilst promoting the APM's values. The five dimensions are breadth, depth, achievement, commitment, and accountability.

The APM has an extensive list of what can be considered formal and informal CPD. Formal CPD includes accredited qualifications, relevant courses, job secondments, conferences, and seminars. Examples of informal CPD can include learning on the job, structured reading, volunteering, and acting as a coach or mentor. The APM also offers an extensive range of qualifications and CPD events covering a variety of skills and topics it deems relevant to the role of Project Manager.

Discussion 3.3

Do you think it is better to have a lower or higher minimum hourly requirement of annual CPD hours?

3.3.4 Institution of Civil Engineers

The Institution of Civil Engineers (ICE) is the professional body for civil engineering in the UK. It supports civil engineers throughout their careers and has more than 95,000 members worldwide. ICE awards professional qualifications that are the industry standard, leads debates around infrastructure and the built environment, and provides an unmatched level of training, knowledge and thinking (ICE, 2020a). ICE has several levels of membership that are explored in more depth in Table 3.11.

Table 3.11 ICE membership levels derived from https://www.ice.org.uk/membership

ICE membership levels	*The authors view of membership levels*
Student Member	Student membership is free and is open to those studying engineering or an engineering-related course at university or college, and also to those working on a placement or apprenticeship.
Graduate Member (GMICE)	Graduate membership is for those with a relevant degree or vocational qualification, who are working towards becoming a professionally qualified civil engineer. ICE refers to the period between academic and professional qualification as 'Initial Professional Development' (IPD). Note that apprentices can join at this grade if they have already gained a relevant academic or vocational qualification.
Technician Member (EngTech MICE)	Technician membership is for those who can apply proven techniques and procedures to the solution of practical engineering problems. To join ICE, you will need to demonstrate your ability and commitment by submitting written evidence, including at least one year of CPD records, and attending an interview.
Member (IEng MICE or CEng MICE)	Membership at incorporated level is for those who maintain and manage applications of current and developing technology, while membership at chartered level is for those who can develop solutions to complex engineering problems through innovation, creativity and technical analysis. To join ICE, you will need to demonstrate your ability and commitment by submitting written evidence, including 3 years' CPD records, and attending a professional review interview and completing a communication task.
Fellow (FICE)	Fellowship is ICE's highest grade of membership, recognising significant contributions made to society and the profession. To join ICE at that level, you will need to provide evidence of meeting the Fellowship attributes and provide 3 years' CPD records to confirm you are leading by example.
Associate Member (AMICE)	Associate membership is open to built environment professionals who want to be part of the civil engineering professional community. To join, you can either show you are a member of a related body or submit a short statement to confirm your interest in civil engineering

3.3.4.1 CPD requirements for the ICE

It is of the authors view that the ICE believes that CPD can be used to evidence a motivation and commitment to career long learning and development. CPD allows members to ensure they stay relevant with up-to-date experience, skills, and knowledge. ICE define CPD as "*The systematic maintenance, improvement and broadening of knowledge and skills, and the development of personal qualities, necessary for the execution of professional and technical duties throughout your working life*" (ICE, 2020b). Continuing professional development (CPD) is a way to show that you are committed to learning and developing throughout your career. To stay relevant, you need to keep your skills, knowledge and experience up to date, record what you learn, and then apply this in your job. As an ICE member, you need to manage your own professional development. If requested to, you should be able to send us an annual record of your past year's CPD.

CPD is undertaken to ensure professionals remain competent. ICE asks its members to think in terms of an annual CPD cycle: reviewing their development needs; planning their CPD; undertaking development activities throughout the year, both planned and taking other development opportunities when they arise; reflecting on their learning; and recording their CPD so they can show that they are maintaining and developing their professional competence. Development action plans and personal development records are discussed in more detail in Chapter 5.

ICE does not set a minimum CPD hours requirement and instead asks its members to do what is required for them to develop and maintain their competence. In practice, the number of CPD hours a member completes will vary based on their registration grade, level of experience, role and responsibility and future career plans. Members generally tend to complete an average of thirty CPD hours a year.

Table 3.12 CPD requirements adapted from ICE membership requirements. Derived from https://www.ice.org.uk/my-ice/membership-documents/continuing-professional-development-guidance

ICE membership levels	*Minimum CPD requirements*
Student	Students on accredited civil engineering courses will be introduced to lifelong learning and they are encouraged to record CPD if they go on work placements.
Graduate Member (GMICE)	Graduate members are expected to undertake CPD each year and they have to submit three CPD records when their 'Initial Professional Development' (IPD) is to be signed-off. Those on an ICE approved training scheme or ICE's mentor supported trainin have access to an online IPD tool to aid their development (ICE, 2021).
Technician Member (EngTech MICE)	Technician Members are expected to undertake CPD each year. They are asked to present one year's CPD records when applying for a professional review and can be asked to submit one year's CPD records as part of ICE's annual CPD audit.
Member (IEng MICE or CEng MICE)	Members are expected to undertake CPD each year. They are asked to present one year's CPD records when applying for a professional review (or three yea if they are applying without having completed their IPD with ICE) and can be asked to submit one year's CPD records as part of ICE's annual CPD audit
Fellow (FICE)	Fellows are expected to undertake CPD each year. They are asked to present three years' CPD records when applying for Fellowship and can be asked to submit one year's CPD records as part of ICE's annual CPD audit.
Associate Member (AMICE)	Associate members are expected to undertake CPD as part of ICE's Code of Professional Conduct.

Discussion 3.4

What are the advantages to reflecting upon your CPD once you have already completed it?

For the most up to date information and guidance on ICE CPD regulations and routes to membership, please visit the ICE website www.ice.org.uk. The ICE has also produced CPD guidance for the different membership grades, which can be seen in Table 3.12 that explains the ongoing CPD requirements and the volume of CPD records reviewed at different assessment stages.

3.3.5 Royal Institute of British Architects

The RIBA is a global body of professional members. It aims to help deliver better buildings, stronger communities, and sustainable environments whilst seeking to drive excellence in architecture. First founded in 1834 the RIBA was awarded a Royal Charter in 1837 and now has over 40,000 global members. There are many pathways to qualify as an Architect; however, an individual must pass the different parts (1, 2, and 3) and gain work experience in order to qualify (RIBA, 2020). Part 1 courses cover the core architectural skills, and there is the chance to gain work experience at stage 1 which follows the completion of part 1. Part 2 courses then provide the individual with enhanced architectural knowledge and again can be followed by practical experience at stage 2. Part 3 is then a further qualification, which the RIBA does provide or other providers can be used. Individuals will then be assessed at a final written and oral examination against their 24 months (minimum) of practical experience, their CV, and a case study they have undertaken. The RIBA has many different membership options available for individuals at different stages of their architecture journey. The authors views of these are described in Table 3.13.

Table 3.13 RIBA membership levels (RIBA, 2020b)

RIBA membership level	*The authors view of the membership levels*
Student Member	Any student on a RIBA-accredited Part 1 or Part 2 course can sign up to be a student member for free and get discounted or free access to a wealth of resources.
Affiliate Member	This level of membership is aimed at those with a professional interest in or passion for architecture. If you are a built environment professional or have a Part 1 qualification, you can gain access to RIBA resources and networks.
Associate Member	This level of membership is exclusive for those with a Part 2 qualification who have gained a professional qualification and have less than two years' experience.
Chartered Member	For those who have achieved Parts 1, 2, and 3, this level of membership is appropriate and you can use the RIBA affix.
Fellow Member	This level of membership recognises those who have made a contribution to the profession of architecture. You can use the FRIBA affix but must be a Chartered Member first and then demonstrate how you have met the criteria outlined by the RIBA as suitable.

3.3.5.1 CPD requirements for the RIBA

It is the authors understanding that all Chartered Members of the RIBA are under an obligation to complete and record 35 hours of annual CPD, with at least half of this classed as 'structured'. The RIBA class structured CPD as having learning aims and outcomes and is formally taught; whereas informal CPD is often conducted alone and of a short duration. The RIBA also has a points-based reflection system for all CPD undertaken. For example, on every CPD event a member attends, they will reflect upon this and assign themselves a score (reflection is covered in more detail in Chapter 6). The scores and descriptions able to be awarded are as follows:

1 If you learnt a little
2 Your general awareness increased through a one- to two-hour activity
3 If you gained a great deal of insight and the activity lasted between half a day and a full day
4 You have acquired expertise and specialist knowledge gained from a course lasting two days or longer

On an annual basis each Chartered Member must achieve 100 points. Out of the 35 hours of annual CPD, 20 hours must also come from the ten mandatory RIBA core curriculum CPD topics, with 2 hours per topic each year (RIBA, 2017). These topics are identified in Table 3.14.

These topics are expanded upon further with a great detailed insight in a RIBA publication entitled 'RIBA CPD Core Curriculum; Continuing Professional Development' (RIBA, 2017). There is an online portal for all Chartered members to record their CPD activities, and the RIBA itself offers courses and programmes that can help all members achieve their CPD requirements, but these are also open to non-members to participate (but who do not receive the discounted member rate).

Discussion 3.5

What are the advantages and disadvantages of using a scoring system when reflecting upon CPD undertaken?

Table 3.14 The authors view of the mandatory RIBA core curriculum CPD topics

• Architecture for social purpose	• Health, safety, and well-being
• Business, clients, and services	• Legal, regulatory, and statutory compliances
• Procurement and contracts	• Sustainable architecture
• Inclusive environments	• Places, planning, and communities
• Building conservation and heritage	• Design, construction, and technology

3.3.6 *Chartered Institute of Procurement and Supply*

The CIPS is a professional body driving the global procurement and supply management profession. It operates across over 150 countries and has over 200,000 members (CIPS, 2020a). Procurement is a major part of the construction industry, and with the ever-increasing role of supply chain managers in companies of all sizes, CIPS as a professional body is becoming more relevant and important in construction with each day. Offering networking opportunities for members, as well as extensive training and development, CIPS has a range of membership levels available. These are explored in more detail in Table 3.15.

3.3.6.1 CPD requirements for the CIPS

CIPS states that CPD is of the upmost importance. It believes that CPD helps develop staff confidence in their own abilities, helps achieve career goals, and enables individuals to successfully respond to change. However, CPD is not mandatory for CIPS members, although it is mandatory if you wish to apply for Chartered Professional Status. CIPS recommends that members should undertake 30 hours annually and have numerous support and guidance documents to help members navigate their CPD requirements (CIPS, 2020b). To assist members in structuring and developing their CPD, CIPS argues that CPD activities can fall into three categories:

1 Knowledge – whereby individuals improve your theoretical and practical knowledge
2 Skills – individuals improving their ability to perform the professional responsibilities required
3 Personal development – where non-procurement-related skills and knowledge are enhanced

Table 3.15 CIPS membership levels

CIPS membership level	*The authors view of membership levels*
Certificate Member	You can become a Certificate Member by achieving level 2 and 3 qualifications.
Diploma Member	A level 4 qualification is required to become a Diploma Member which can be gained from CIPS or the completion of the first year of a traditional three-year university degree course.
Associate Member	A level 5 qualification allows individuals to become an Associate Member.
Full Member (MCIPS)	Full membership of CIPS is only achieved with the completion of an applicable level 6 qualification and three years' work experience.
Fellow (FCIPS)	You must be an MCIPS and be either a senior procurement professional or a leading procurement consultant or academic, and driven to promote the profession.

CIPS has online facilities for members to record their CPD and has lengthy guidance on what activities constitute fall into each of the three CPD activity categories. These can include e-learning and reading, with every hour spent reading able to be recorded as one hour of CPD; mentoring and conference attendance, with again every hour spent on such activities worth an hour of CPD; and also gaining non-CIPS qualifications which are classed as professional development and are worth up to 30 CPD hours per qualification gained.

To ensure compliance with its CPD requirements, the CIPS randomly audits members. The CIPS also requires a learning statement to be in place when undertaking CPD. This is a written document that allows reflection on any learning undertaken to occur. This should help members consider how any CPD activity has had a positive impact on their personal and professional abilities and ensure that CPD activities undertaken are done so with an expected learning outcome in mind.

3.3.7 *Institute of Chartered Accountants England and Wales*

The ICAEW is a professional body for those in the accountancy and finance professions. It has over 154,000 professional members across 148 countries and has been in existence since its formation in 1880. This is a professional body that operates across many industries, including construction, as the construction industry does have many accountancy and financial management staff working at companies of all sizes. To qualify as a Chartered Accountant, individuals must complete the Associate Chartered Accountant (ACA) requirements. This is a process that consists of gaining 450 days of professional work experience, passing 15 exam modules, demonstrating transparency and abidance by the ICAEW code of ethics, and evidencing professional development in seven core areas (ICAEW, 2017). These core areas are as follows:

1. Adding value
2. Communication
3. Decision-making
4. Ethics and professionalism
5. Problem-solving
6. Teamwork
7. Technical competence

3.3.7.1 CPD requirements for the ICAEW

The ICAEW requires members to make a CPD declaration every year. This is the procedure to formally confirm you have undertaken the required annual CPD. There is no need to upload the CPD records you have kept, but records should be maintained in a case you are required to submit them if you are one of the members who are randomly selected each month to have their CPD records reviewed.

There is no formal CPD annual hour requirement for each member to undertake; however, the ICAEW recommends that all members should adopt the following approach when undertaking their CPD requirements (ICAEW, 2020):

- Reflect – consider development needs and your changing role and aim to build on any knowledge gaps you have identified.
- Act – undertake relevant CPD activities including online learning, workshops, meetings, reading, and conferences.
- Impact – assess the effectiveness of the activities undertaken against any knowledge gaps identified. Consider if the activity has made you more competent and improved your ability.

3.4 Overlapping CPD requirements

There are also many more professional bodies operating in the construction industry and related fields. These include the Chartered Association of Building Engineers (CABE) and the Chartered Institute of Architectural Technologists (CIAT) that both require all their respective members to undertake 35 hours of annual CPD (CABE, 2020; CIAT, 2020). The Chartered Institute of Civil Engineering Surveyors (CICES) has no annual hour obligations, but does have a CPD policy that requires all members to undertake appropriate CPD to maintain and improve professional competence (CICES, 2020). The Chartered Institute of Personnel and Development (CIPD) has over 150,000 members and adopts a similar approach of having no annual hour CPD requirements, but does expect members to undertake quality CPD activities that result in useful experiences and practical benefits (CIPD, 2020).

We can see from the different professional bodies reviewed in this chapter that the one thing they all have in common is the need for their members to undertake some form of CPD on an annual basis. These CPD requirements do differ in terms of annual hours required to be recorded, and sometimes in what is considered informal and formal CPD – but the principles of self-development remain the same. It is therefore possible to be a member of numerous professional bodies simultaneously and satisfy each of the CPD requirements by undertaking one set of activities. A comparison of the professional body CPD requirements also reveals that members need to take responsibility for their own development and undertake a process of goal identification and setting (explored in Chapter 4), goal planning and the completion of activities (explored in Chapter 5), and also a process of self-reflection (explored in Chapter 6). Table 3.16 highlights some of the key CPD requirements of the professional bodies summarised in this chapter.

Table 3.16 Key Professional Body CPD requirements

Key Professional Body CPD Requirements
1 Ensure you have a recorded CPD plan of what you want to achieve and by when
2 This can and should include a varied mixture of formal and informal CPD activities
3 You can categorise CPD activities to ensure they are relevant, either directly or indirectly, to your current or future role
4 CPD activities need to be identified and considered before undertaking, and then reflected upon post completion (including potential scoring).
5 Beware of all standards set for the quality and quantity of CPD you are required to undertake annually

3.5 Professional body rules and non-members

It is also worth noting that even if you are not a member of a professional body and have no intention of becoming one, you should still undertake the same rigorous CPD requirements. There are numerous reasons for this, some of which are explored below:

First, the importance of CPD extends far beyond professional body requirements. In order to become and remain competent at our day-to-day responsibilities, we must all ensure we are suitably trained and have the required skill set. As all roles are also evolving with the onset of technology, innovative practices, and simply more efficiency as tasks are repeated, we also must ensure our knowledge evolves too. CPD is an ideal way, if not the only way, we can ensure our skill sets remain relevant in an increasingly changing industry.

Second, whilst you may not be held to account by a professional body regarding your CPD if you are not a member, you will certainly be held to account by your employer, and perhaps even a third party tasked with resolving a dispute if you are ever involved in one. If the leading professional body in your particular profession has released best practice guidance on a certain issue, then you need to be aware of it, and if you do not follow that guidance, and those actions ultimately lead to a dispute, then your actions and ultimately your competency and professionalism will be scrutinised. Therefore, it will be your CPD that is being challenged, and questions asked regarding your professional development, such as:

- Have you made conscious efforts to be up to date with what is required of someone in your role?
- Did you then act in a way that is considered the most appropriate and correct?

Maintaining CPD is the best way to ensure your skill sets, knowledge, and abilities remain high, ensuring you can deliver high levels of professional standards and quality in all tasks that you undertake.

3.5 Conclusion

This chapter introduced the concept of professional bodies. These are organisations that usually sit within a single profession or industry and consist of individual members who aim to promote best practices and set the standards and expectations of behaviour for both their own members and the wider profession and industry. There are many professional bodies that operate within the construction industry. Some operate solely within the industry, whilst others operate solely for a particular profession that may span several industries. This chapter covers only a few of the professional bodies that operate within the construction industry; there are many more that are relevant and that could be more applicable to your particular role and career plan. This chapter does explore the professional bodies in some detail and focuses upon the individual body's CPD requirements and expectations of their members. We can see that the RICS requires its members to complete and record 20 hours of CPD per year, with 10 of those needing to be formal. Other professional bodies, such the APM and RIBA, require 35 hours of CPD to be recorded, whilst the CIOB and ICE do not set formal annual hourly minimum CPD requirements for their members to achieve, but instead encourage members to complete as much CPD as they feel relevant to their role and current development needs.

Ultimately however, all professional bodies do require CPD of members, and whether you are a current member or have no intention of becoming a member of a professional body, it is advisable to engage with CPD requirements to ensure your knowledge, skills, and experience remain up to date and relevant in an ever-changing and increasingly demanding industry.

3.6 Discussion Answers

Discussion 3.1: What are the advantages and disadvantages of having a set minimum annual CPD hour requirement? The advantages to having a set amount of required CPD hours include the assurance that each professional body member is achieving a certain level of development each year. However, there is no guarantee over the quality of that COD. By not having a set amount of annual CPD hours required, members are free to focus on fewer more appropriate CPD activities. However, this could be open to abuse and some professionals and organisations may not realise the importance of CPD, especially during busy periods at work.

Discussion 3.2: What are the advantages and disadvantages of having no set minimum annual CPD requirements? As introduced in the above, having no quantitative CPD requirements can be freeing in that it allows individuals to focus on the CPD they feel is most applicable to their role and future career development. Professionals are then somewhat free from scrutiny in deciding if a CPD activity is suitable and do not need to sign up to events that they may have little personal interest and little professional gain simply to achieve a set number of hours. However, without having a set amount of annual CPD hours to record, a professional's time may be monopolised by immediate work commitments (as it so often is in the construction industry) and they may go long periods of time without giving suitable consideration to their CPD. Having an annual CPD commitment they are required to undertake can serve as a productive and timely reminder that development is of high importance.

Discussion 3.3: Do you think it Is better to have a lower or higher minimum hourly requirement of annual CPD hours? Different professional bodies take different approaches to the number of hours their members are required. Some are higher than others. If you do have set requirements with regards to the amount of CPD hours you are required to undertake and record on an annual basis, you may think these are too low or overly high when compared to other professional body requirements. In short, there is no right or wrong number of CPD hours to record annually. The advantages of having to record more of that more CPD is ultimately undertaken, whereas a disadvantage is that these CPD hours may simply be undertaken to meet the requirements and with little consideration given to their practical use. Having a lower number of CPD hours to record may allow professionals to focus on development opportunities they feel most relevant but may equally not set the threshold of hours to achieve high enough for the development needs of some professionals. As the hourly requirements are set by the respective professional body, if you want to gain membership, and then continue to be a member, it is important you are aware of the annual CPD hourly requirements and that these are achieved. Although somewhat regardless of the hourly requirements, it is the quality of CPD undertaken that is key.

Discussion point 3.4: What are the advantages to reflecting upon your CPD once you have already completed it?

Some may think once CPD is completed it is simply a matter of recording the activity and then moving on – to either the next CPD activity or back to work not to have to think about CPD again until the next time. However, it is only by reflecting upon CPD (explored more in Chapter 6) that it is truly understood, key lessons are identified and considered in greater depth, and the type of activity itself can be analysed for it's successes and failures to help you better plan future CPD activities.

Discussion 3.5: What are the advantages and disadvantages of using a scoring system when reflecting upon CPD undertaken?

Some form of reflection is better than no reflection. However, conducting a detailed and robust reflection of CPD activities undertaken is ideal to really understand not just the main lessons of the activity itself, but the other insights you may have gained. Having a formal scoring mechanism will also remove elements of subjectivity when reflecting upon the CPD activity and ensure that you can objectively monitor and record what occurred, what you learnt, if it was effective and how it will contribute to your future development. It will also allow you to see (when compared against set criteria and thresholds) if the CPD activities you are undertaking are meeting the requirements set (either by yourself, your employer or a professional body). A potential downside to scoring as part of any reflection is that a CPD activity you may really enjoy, or believe you will gain a lot from, may be overlooked if it does not meet the immediate criteria of achieving a high score.

References

APM (2020a). *APM Code of Professional Conduct.* Available from: https://www.apm.org.uk/about-us/how-apm-is-run/apm-code-of-professional-conduct/

APM (2020b). *About CPD.* Available from: https://www.apm.org.uk/cpd/about-cpd/

APM (2020c). *Inspiring Positive Change.* Available from: https://www.apm.org.uk/news/inspiring-positive-change/

CABE (2020). *Continuing Professional Development.* Available from: https://cbuilde.com/page/cpd

CIAT (2020). *What Is CPD?* Available from: https://ciat.org.uk/education/cpd/continuing-professional-development.html

CICES (2020). *CPD.* Available from: https://www.cices.org/membership/about/cpd/

CIOB (2015). *Professionalism and Integrity in Construction; Code of Professional Conduct and Rules.* Available from: https://www.ciob.org/sites/default/files/Code%20of%20Conduct%20for%20Chartered%20Building%20Consultancies_0.pdf

CIOB (2018). *Rules and Regulations of Professional Competence and Conduct.* Available from: https://www.ciob.org/sites/default/files/Rules%20and%20Regulation%20of%20Professional%20Competence%20and%20Conduct.pdf

CIOB (2020). *About Us.* Available from: https://www.ciob.org/about#:~:text=The%20Chartered%20Institute%20of%20Building%20is%20at%20the%20heart%20of,for%20construction%20management%20and%20leadership.

CIPD (2020). *Continuing Professional Development.* Available from: https://www.cipd.co.uk/learn/cpd

CIPS (2020a). *What Is CIPS Membership?* Available from: https://www.cips.org/membership/cips-membership/

CIPS (2020b). *Continuing Professional Development.* Available from: https://www.cips.org/membership/benefits-of-membership/cpd/

ICAEW (2017). ICAEW Professional development skills. Available from: https://www.icaew.com/learning-and-development/campaigns/professional-skills-update/skills

ICAEW (2020). Our guide to CPD. Available from: https://www.icaew.com/membership/cpd/what-is-cpd/our-guide-to-cpd

ICE (2020a). *Our Mission and Work.* Available from: https://www.ice.org.uk/about-ice/governance/our-mission-and-work#:~:text=We%20aim%20to%20be%3A,built%20environment%20around%20the%20world.&text=The%20professional%20engineering%20association%20that,help%20in%20tackling%20global%20challenges

ICE (2020b). *Continuing Professional Development.* Available from: https://www.ice.org.uk/my-ice/my-membership/continuing-professional-development

ICE (2021) ICE Training Scheme Guidance. Available from: https://www.ice.org.uk/my-ice/membership-documents/ice-training-scheme

IES-C (2016). *International Ethics Standards. An Ethical Framework for the Global Property Market.* Available from: https://ricstest.files.wordpress.com/2016/12/international-ethics-standards-final.pdf

RIBA (2017). *RIBA CPD Core Curriculum.* Available from: https://www.architecture.com/-/media/files/CPD/CPD-Core-Curriculum/RIBA-CPD-Core-Curriculum-2018.pdf

RIBA (2020). *Our History, Charter and Byelaws.* Available from: https://www.architecture.com/about/history-charter-and-byelaws

RIBA (2020b). Join the RIBA. Available from: ihttps://www.architecture.com/join-riba

RICS (2020a). *About Us.* Available from: https://www.rics.org/uk/about-rics/?link=useful-links&_ga=2.113475207.1053517847.1600258551-268095219.1600258551

RICS (2020b). *Rules of Conduct for Members. Version 7 with Effect from 2 March 2020.* Available from: https://www.rics.org/globalassets/rics-website/media/upholding-professional-standards/regulation/rules-of-conduct-for-members_2020.pdf

RICS (2020c). *Rules of Conduct for Firms. Version 7 with Effect from 2 March 2020.* Available from: https://www.rics.org/globalassets/rics-website/media/upholding-professional-standards/regulation/rules-of-conduct-for-firms_2020.pdf

RICS (2020d). *CPD Compliance Guide.* Available from: https://www.rics.org/uk/upholding-professional-standards/regulation/cpd-compliance-guide/

4 Goal setting

4.1 Introduction

This chapter discusses how and why goals are set. It is the setting of goals that facilitates personal and professional development. Whilst organisations can set any goals for their employees they feel are appropriate, these will almost always be linked to immediate financial returns for the company. This is not a negative idea per se but can often stifle individual's own development plans and may lead to a reduction in external opportunities. This is not to say people should not engage with the development opportunities offered as it is always a great idea to embrace any development opportunity available. However, individual's need to be aware that employer offered development may only develop employees for current and future roles of the company and the skills may not be transferable. It is therefore of the upmost importance that individuals take responsibility for their own development. Understanding how to set clear and focused goals, and then how to dissect and analyse these goals so the constituent parts can be explored, planned, and achieved is key. A range of methods for setting goals is explored in this chapter, as are skills and techniques for understanding how to break such goals down into manageable steps. Several analysis methods, such as SWOT, SMART, FAST, and STEEPLE, are explored and how these can be applied to goal setting is discussed. The aim of this chapter is to understand how clear, focused, and effective goals are set as this will increase the likelihood they can and will be successfully achieved.

4.2 What are goals?

A goal can be described as the object of an individual's ambition. A target or objective that they can set for themselves can set in conjunction with someone else (i.e. colleagues or family) or that someone else can set on their behalf (i.e. management). This can include both personal and professional targets, and both are of equal importance to well-balanced development. Whilst terminology can be interchanged and definitions overlap, in this textbook we will use the term 'goal' to define the overall and ultimate aim an individual seeks to achieve. The term 'milestones' will be used to describe the smaller goals and intermittent steps or objectives an individual accomplishes on their way to achieve their overall goal.

Example 4.1

A trainee Quantity Surveyor (QS) may set themselves the goal of becoming Chartered with the RICS. In order to do so, they will have to complete many milestones on their way to achieve this goal including recording the required amount of experience, attending formal CPD courses, and completing and submitting their diaries and reports on their competency knowledge. Each of these would be considered an milestone to be completed on their way to achieve their overall goal – without the completion of an milestone, the goal would not be achieved.

4.3 Why set goals?

The literature on why we should set goals is vast. The benefits have been widely explored. Such benefits include an increase in motivation; you are more likely to be willing to commit your time and effort to something if that something is clear in your mind and is a goal you have set yourself to achieve. An increase in focus is another benefit from goal setting; you are able to focus and commit energy to a task if it is set, and you can foresee the benefits completion of the task will bring. Setting goals also helps with self-organisation; being aware of a goal enables you to structure your life accordingly, so you can dedicate the amount of time required to satisfy its completion. Ultimately, the setting of a goal will allow you to monitor and track your progress against achieving the goal. Witnessing progress towards a goal, which is helped with regular monitoring, will in turn mean the goal feels more within reach and help set expectations so you know when the goal can be achieved, and not to be hard on yourself and lose motivation if you feel it is not happening sooner than it ever realistically could.

4.4 Goal selection

Selecting a goal to focus your energy and effort on for some may seem a simple and straight forward step that takes minimal time and is easy to complete. For others selecting a goal can be seen the single biggest step that takes the longest time to consider and execute correctly. It is a combination of these methods that is most successfully employed when it comes to the setting of goals, with different techniques required for different purposes and in different circumstances. Both methods are explored in more detail below, discussed as quick goal setting (QGS) and insightful goal setting.

4.4.1 Quick goal setting

Quick goal setting (QGS) has a very important place in an individual's development. Not all goals need to be lifelong dreams or considered with such insight that days and weeks are spent agonising over their every detail almost to the point of paralysis. In fact, if you find you are stuck in such a situation, you may discover that QGS actually helps you successfully escape such as a rut.

QGS is precisely that. It is the setting of generally smaller goals that require less undertaking to be completed. These can be steps either directly or indirectly linked to the achievement of longer term goals or can be one-off and stand-alone goals. The goals set as part of a QGS exercise can be based on any number of criteria. Several potential criteria are listed in Table 4.1.

The list of criteria is by no means exhaustive, and neither are they meant to be considered in isolation. Often decisions will be made based on a multiple of these factors. The purpose of QGS is to identify (and take advantage of) opportunities that you would not automatically think of. Such opportunities may then lead to new unexpected ideas and areas for development. You may also find lessons learnt and ideas generated can also be transferred to other aspects of your professional life. Solutions for long-standing problems you were once stuck may be more forthcoming, and innovative methods improving on current practices may be developed.

The completion of 'quick goals' can help improve motivation, which can then be directed at larger goals. Completion of such goals can also help improve happiness and general life satisfaction as well as mental well-being. QGS can also include goals that are long-term professional targets and can always be items that will benefit your immediate role or future career progression directly. It is

Table 4.1 Potential QGS criteria

QGS criteria	*Description*
Cost	You may only have a fixed budget available from either savings or a work-based training and development fund. Therefore, you can start a search for development opportunities that fit this budget.
Time	You may have a week's holiday, have a longer career break, have recently retired, or only have one evening a week to commit. But knowing your time restraints beforehand can help you identify suitable opportunities for development that easily fit around your current lifestyle.
Location	You may be moving to a temporary location for work for a set period of time, relocating on a more permanent basis, or not have the means to travel very far from where you are currently based. Identifying courses based on location increases the chances of successful completion.
Qualification	Sometimes the completion of a course can lead to more than CPD credits to meet any professional requirement. The successful completion of some courses results in a qualification that is often widely recognised.
End use	The course or development opportunity may result in a practical end use where you can immediately apply the knowledge you have learnt to your own situation for professional gain.
Ease of completion	You may want a relaxing challenge during a week off or a more in-depth commitment that will increase your focus and sense of achievement.

unfortunate, however, that some people fail to see the benefit of QGS when they are not immediately linked to a current role. As a method of achieving immediate- and short-term success whilst ultimately lead to the accomplishment of long-term goals, QGS can be an invaluable technique.

4.4.2 Insightful goal setting

Whilst QSP does have numerous benefits, insightful well-thought out goals are often the ones that spring to mind when people discuss goal setting. For the purpose of discussion, this textbook breaks such goals into those that can be considered short-term, medium-term, and long-term. The time frames associated with each type of goal are purely at the discretion of the goal setter, or in the case of line management involvement, as the result of a discussion between the goal setter and the individual working towards achieving the goal. Either way insightful goals are the ones that we strive to achieve and the ones we think about, dream about, the goals that require a degree of planning and forethought.

Ultimately any goal is achievable with detailed planning to break down goals into smaller achievable steps. The old adage of how do you eat an elephant is the perfect metaphor for goal planning – but before you can plan to achieve a goal, you need to set it. Goals can be set as short-, medium-, or long-term. By classing a goal into one of these categories, it can help you realise how achievable the goal is, or perhaps how unachievable it is in the short term, and help you to place a realistic time frame on achievement to help manage your own expectations and those around you; but ultimately you achieve the long-term goals in much the same way as you eat an elephant – one bite at a time.

4.4.3 Short-term goals

Short-term goals can be those you wish to achieve today, this week, month, or year. You could stretch out your boundaries to cover a longer period if you wanted, or if set by your organisation. Short-term goals can be milestones on the way to achieve medium-term or longer term goal or can themselves be the ultimate goals you aim to achieve. Inevitably some goals will start as long-term goals, and as progression is made and time passes, they will become medium-term goals and then ultimately short-term goals. Short-term goals are the ones that should have the most clarity and the ones that should be prepared for and completed first. These are goals that have plans in place to achieve and ones that have been considered the most. For example, if we take becoming a Chartered Member of a construction-related professional body, you will be able to clearly break down the steps required to achieve this goal into time-related segments, with key milestones identified. You may have identified the need to register as a member within the next month, and then give yourself three months to complete the application, with a further two months for the professional body to respond and arrange an interview. Therefore, your goal of becoming chartered could be achieved within the next six months, and you have clear steps that need to be completed to make it happen. Breaking down goals in such a manner will allow them to be suitably classed as short, medium, or long-term to allow everyone's expectations to be managed effectively. You would not, however, record your short-term goals in the manner done so above as this would not be conducive to making any changes to the goals or monitoring and updating progress. Chapter 5 considers effective methods of recording goals, milestones, and how to generally develop and present professional development plans.

4.4.4 *Medium-term goals*

Medium-term goals will have their own time frames. These will be goals that are not achievable in the short term due to the steps required to achieve them and/or the duration that they take to accomplish. However, such goals will be achievable before other goals which are classed as long-term goals. Medium-term goals, as you imagine due to their location between short- and long-term goals, will not have as much detail as short-term goals with regard to the steps required to complete, but you will have a broad plan in place to achieve them at some point. Figure 4.2 shows broadly the level of detail medium-term goals will have in comparison with short-term and long-term goals. However, rather than being simply a transition space where long-term goals become short-term goals, medium-term goals allow us to dedicate more time and focus, and act as an important stage in how we change our perceptions of the goals we are wanting to achieve. If long-term goals represent more 'blue sky thinking' in that they are optimistic and challenging, when goals become medium-term, a greater level of focus and attention needs to be paid to them. This includes mapping out the key milestones we need to undertake to bring the goal closer to achievement, ensuring we remain on track to achieve the goal by the date planned and start to consider what resources we may need and any problems we may encounter. An example of a medium-term goal could be the promotion from Assistant Project Manager (APM) to a Project Manager (PM) role. If you are relatively new in your role of APM, you wouldn't expect a promotion to PM to occur in the short term, but having this as a medium-term goal is realistic. Whilst you may not have a detailed plan in place to achieve the promotion right now, as it is a medium-term goal you should have broad career steps in mind to achieve it such as complete your current project, register with a professional body, complete relevant work-based training courses on specialised software, shadow colleagues, and discuss the promotion with your existing line manager.

4.4.5 *Long-term goals*

Long-term goals do not require detailed milestones in place. You do not need to even consider exactly when long-term goals will be achieved; approximate years of completion will suffice. Long-term goals act as a direction of travel, a horizon you aim for. You will align your medium- and short-term goals accordingly to

Table 4.2 Short-, medium-, and long-term goal details

Short-term goals	These goals should be clear, with detailed steps in place that are all achievable within a set time frame.
Medium-term goals	These goals can be major milestones on the way to achieving longer term goals or end goals themselves that are not quite achievable in the immediate short term.
Long-term goals	These goals can be less well defined and more approximate. They may not be clear and may simply be vague roles or careers that you would like to explore.

ensure you are focused towards your long-term goals, and be aware of the broad stages you will need to follow, but generally you will not focus on the long-term goals themselves on a daily basis. However, having a long-term goal in mind will help increase your focus and motivation, knowing that with each short-term and medium-term goals achieved, you are one step closer to achieving any long-harboured ambitions. Having long-term goals in place can also make you more resilient to short-term setbacks, and also more willing to suffer short-term difficulties. If you know something (such as a current role within a team or current company you are employed by) will not last forever, but will inevitably lead to something better, and something that you have listed as a medium- or long-term goal, you are more likely to endure the short-term hardship. For example, starting your own consultancy may be something you dream of doing, and so set as your long-term goal. Whilst this goal should drive you forward and aid motivation, it will not be something you explicitly think of everyday, but it will inform your short-term goals in that you may wish to gain as much experience of one work environment as you can, and then look to move elsewhere to broaden your business experience. You may also plan to move into a more client-focused role in the medium term to improve your negotiation and work winning communication abilities (Table 4.2).

4.5 Milestones

In terms of goal setting, in this textbook milestones are intermittent steps, or mini goals, that will be accomplished in the progress of achieving a wider goal. Short-term goals can be used as milestones to map and monitor progress against medium- and long-term goals. Consideration should be given to milestones, as they need to represent the steps that you forecast it will take to progress towards the identified goal. The process of identifying milestones should start after the identification of a goal. Once a goal is identified, an exercise should be undertaken whereby the goal is analysed and broken down into smaller constituent parts. These parts should then be arranged into a consistent and chronological order. This will then provide a structure of milestones against which progress towards a desired goal can be measured. Practical examples of this technique and more methods of goal monitoring and CPD Plan structuring can be found in Chapter 5.

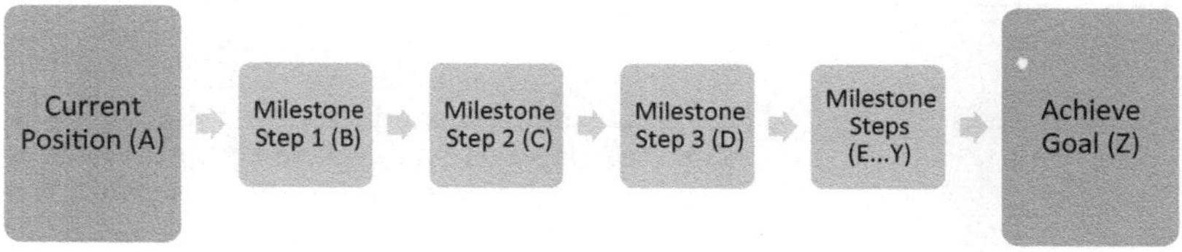

Figure 4.1 Milestones in Goal Setting.

Milestones should be considered as the journey from current position to end goal. If you are currently at 'A', your end goal is 'Z'. Each letter of the alphabet in between can be considered a milestone step. Making each milestones short and simple is an effective practice. Having a milestone that is complex and very difficult can prove problematic as individuals can become stuck on a single milestone for a long period of time, making it appear that progress is not being made against goal achievement. If milestones are broken down into small simple steps, each step can be achieved relatively simply, thereby showing the progress that is being made whilst maintaining and enhancing motivation. Considering goals in great detail to identify milestones can also reveal steps required that were not initially identified and so allow a greater level of goal analysis to occur. The more that is known about the requirements of a goal, the more likely that goal will ultimately be achieved.

4.6 Goal-setting theory

In the journal *Organisational Behaviour and Human Performance* published in 1968, an American psychologist called Edwin Locke was part of a team that published an article proposing the idea that would go on to become goal-setting theory (GST). In the article Locke sought to examine the relationship between conscious goal setting, individual intentions towards achieving the goal, and the task performance itself. Locke went on to summarise that the harder the goal set, the higher the level of performance. He also argued that the more specific the goal, the higher the level of output produced and that behavioural intentions regulate choice behaviour. Locke's GST goes on to state that monetary incentives and imposed time limits do not have an impact on performance levels independently of goals and intentions – it is an individual's conscious goal and intentional choices that motivate them to complete the goal to the highest level they can.

Concluding his original paper, Locke argues that the goals themselves and the intentions of individuals are key determinants of task performance. In order for incentives to impact behaviour, an individual will need to recognise and evaluate the incentive and develop goals and intentions in response to their evaluation. Locke's paper then suggests the following sequence to hypothesise how environmental events lead to action.

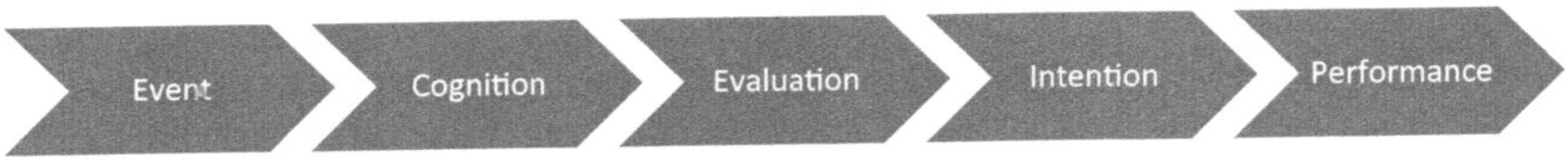

Figure 4.2 Adapted from Locke's goal-setting theory derived from Locke, et al., (1986).

Whilst Locke's theory was just that – a theory, it does have applications to real-world settings. Although it could be argued that employees do not often have the opportunity to set their own goals, individuals can still utilise GST when understanding their own goal-setting and goal-achieving behaviour. Ultimately, by setting specific and ambitious goals, higher performance is often exhibited in order to achieve the goals set.

4.7 Goal-setting practice

When it comes actually considering what you want to achieve, and any goals you want to set yourself, or perhaps goals you will be setting for other people, there are many techniques and tools that can be employed to assist you in ensuring you set successful goals. This may seem obvious, or perhaps a step that you have never considered before, and whilst there are no incorrect goals themselves, by setting a goal incorrectly you can make it much harder to achieve than it needed to be. One method that can help you set clear and coherent goals is the conducting of a SWOT analysis.

4.7.1 SWOT analysis

SWOT is an acronym for strengths, weaknesses, opportunities, and threats. A SWOT analysis is a reflective tool used by both individuals and organisations to identify their own characteristics and help forward planning. Quite simply a SWOT analysis is an exercise undertaken either alone or in a group whereby elements of a particular idea, aspect, characteristic, project, etc. are analysed against the four categories. Figure 4.3 illustrates the form a SWOT analysis may take:

Strengths	**Weaknesses**
Opportunities	**Threats**

Figure 4.3 SWOT Analysis.

As an example, for an idea you have you will identify and list all the strengths of the idea you can think of, all of the weaknesses that may hold it back, all of the opportunities available for help developing and launching the idea, and any external threats that could limit the idea's potential for success. As a broad rule for populating a SWOT analysis, the strengths and weaknesses are considered internal factors with opportunities and threats considered external. Internal are all the elements that are personal to you as an individual, whereas external are the company, industry, and sector-wide aspects that you may be able to take advantage of or that may serve as a broader threat to your professional development and wider career.

It should be noted that you may be aware of concepts under different names or the same concept but with different titles, such as examples where 'weaknesses' are substituted for the more positive 'areas to be developed'. The use of any similar concepts or changes to the SWOT analysis is acceptable; it is the process of reflection and ultimate aim of goal identification that is important. In relation to professional development and the goal setting of an individual, there are two main ways of implementing a SWOT analysis. The first is to identify a goal, and the second is to help achieve a goal.

4.7.1.1 SWOT analysis to identify a goal

Once a reflective SWOT analysis is undertaken, you may decide to identify and set a goal based on an assessment of the opportunities available. The completion of the SWOT will help reveal any opportunities, and by conducting the SWOT analysis with help from others, you may find opportunities available you never initially realised. These opportunities may then form part of your QGS practice or may become medium-term goals as they may take some preparatory work or the accomplishment of milestones in order to begin.

Any threats identified as part of your reflective SWOT may also lead to the development of goals. This could be in relation to immediate events or events forecast to occur longer term, for example, if you identify new software you are unfamiliar with, but that is being increasingly used in your company and amongst competitors. The threat could be an immediate reduction in the number of projects you can work on, or longer term it could mean a lack of career opportunities available. You can therefore use this threat as a goal; to get training and experience on the software so the anticipated threats are never experienced.

Whilst identification of your strengths may not initially feel like it helps identify potential goals, you need to ensure the strengths you have, and are perceived to have, are maintained. If you have a lack of experience in an area and this is well known, then the expectations placed on you within your organisation should take this into account. However, if you are perceived as an expert on a particular topic, then it is arguably more important that your skills are maintained and enhanced. For example, if you have expert knowledge of the NEC3, then you will be viewed as an expert in this area; however, if you failed to update your knowledge when the NEC4 suite of contracts was released, you will be unable to advise people with the same degree of expertise, and any perceptions colleagues had of your expertise may soon begin to fade.

The weaknesses identified as part of a reflective SWOT analysis are probably by far the easiest way of identifying appropriate goals. If you have identified a weakness in your knowledge, experience, or ability, setting this as a goal is an easy way to develop and to evidence your development. This can be beneficial if you are utilising QGS or if you want to generally improve in areas you honestly feel are important and you are lacking the required competence. Numerous professional bodies throughout the construction industry have an obligation for members to act within their competence (see Chapter 3), and so ensuring you are competent for any task ahead is of paramount importance to abide by professional body requirements. Wider than professional body requirements, however, is the need to be competent to carry out required tasks, even if there is no obligation compelling you to stay abreast of professional developments. This is to ensure you can be counted on by your colleagues and clients, and to know you can count on them in a mutually trusting and productive environment.

An example of how a SWOT analysis can help identify a goal, or goals, to achieve can be seen in Figure 4.4. In this example, a Graduate QS in their first year of employment at a consultancy is reflecting upon their own abilities in order to identify professional development goals.

In the above example, the Graduate QS may identify their current presentation skills as an immediate weakness to develop and so look for training courses in this area ranging from online taster sessions, more formal CPD events, or even specifically focused training courses. The weakness of limited project experience may lead to the goal of 'gaining project experience'. The opportunity of experienced colleagues may help achieve this goal as by discussing with colleagues, they may allow you to visit their projects and shadow them during meetings, and once they are aware of your motivation and enthusiasm, they may get you directly involved in the completion of tasks. The weakness of low confidence could be linked to the maximising of other opportunities. If the Graduate QS begins the journey to become a Chartered QS, this could increase their employability and promotion

Strengths	**Weaknesses**
• Achieved University Degree • Enthusiastic and highly motivated • Good IT skills	• Limited project experience • Poor presentation skills • Low office confidence
Opportunities	**Threats**
• Many colleagues to learn from • Further formal and informal study • Can start journey to Chartered professional	• Competition for promotions from colleagues • Economic performance of construction industry may go down resulting in redundancies

Figure 4.4 SWOT Analysis to help identify goals.

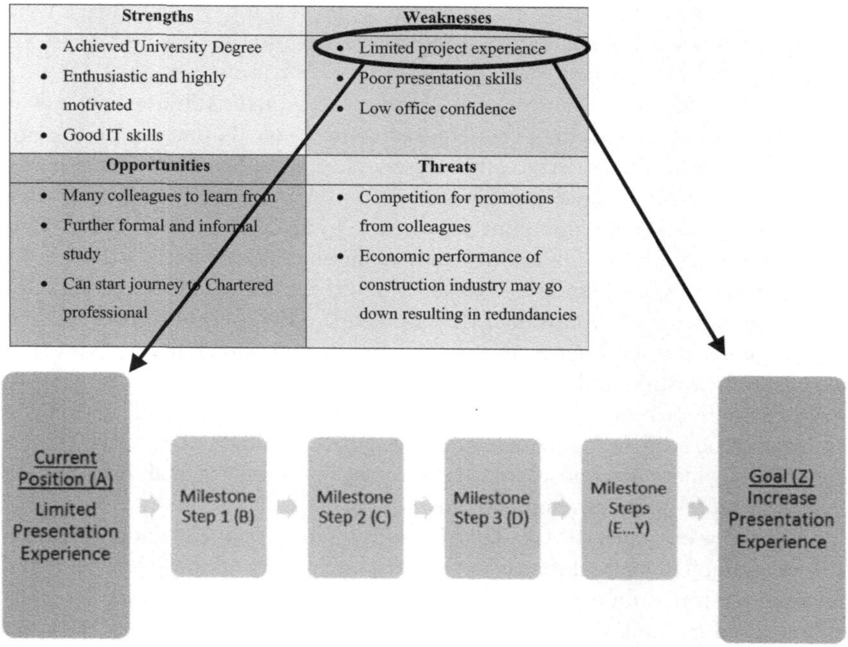

Figure 4.5 SWOT as a goal setting tool.

opportunities and reduce chances of redundancy, thereby potentially improving professional confidence.

4.7.1.2 SWOT analysis to help achieve a goal

If you have a goal in mind already, regardless of if it is a short-, medium-, or long-term goal, then conducting a SWOT analysis on that particular goal, instead of on yourself generally, can help create a plan of how you can achieve the goal. A correctly conducted SWOT analysis can reveal elements linked to a goal's achievement you may not initially have associated with the goal and can allow you to focus your effort on aspects directly and indirectly linked to achieving the goal analysed.

For example, if the goal you have in mind is to find employment elsewhere, but at a higher position, say from QS to Senior QS (SQS). Utilising a SWOT analysis with a specific focus on your skills and experience in relation to the goal of promotion, rather than a SWOT analysis of your skills and experience in general, would enable a tailored and focus approach to how you can achieve this specific goal. It will consider your current strengths in relation to a promotion and performing at a senior level and what weaknesses you have that you will need to address, such as interview practice and people management skills. The SWOT analysis would also allow you to identify any opportunities for development such as online interview resources and CPD courses related to management. Finally, the SWOT analysis could help identify any threats that may stand in the way of you achieving your goal of promotion, and by identifying such threats you can develop plans to tackle, mitigate, or avoid them where possible. Figure 4.6 provides an example of how a SWOT analysis can be applied to a specific goal. In this example, we will consider the same gradate QS as before, but this time they are reflecting upon, and specifically populating the SWOT analysis with factors relating to the goal of becoming a Chartered QS.

In this example, the SWOT analysis has been utilised around a specific goal to better help understand how that goal can be successfully achieved. The information the analysis reveals can then be acted upon to create the milestones that need to be completed in order for the overall goal to be reached. The weakness of a poor interview technique can be addressed through the use of online courses and practice interviews with colleagues undergoing the same route to Chartered status. The threat of potential changes on time demands can be mitigated by the completion of many activities possible in the short term where available time as a resource is a strength. Not all elements identified can be mitigated or taken advantage of; in this instance, this could be the threat of redundancy. This may not be something that can be specifically addressed in the performance of this goal, but is just a factor to be aware of, that serves to enhance the overall motivation to complete the goal in a timely manner whilst the opportunities exist.

In the examples described above, SWOT analysis is simply a tool to help identify goals and to help break the identified goals down into personalised detail to better understand how they can be achieved. SWOT analysis is not always needed to do this but can always serve as a reminder of best practice. Once goals are

Strengths	**Weaknesses**
• Awareness of current QS role requirements • Lots of time to dedicate to the process after work • Enthusiasm to become Chartered	• Lack of understanding of some concepts • Not very organised • Poor interview technique
Opportunities	**Threats**
• Lots of Chartered professionals at current office • Colleagues undergoing same process simultaneously • Online resources and course available	• Time demands may change if I gain promotion • Limited opportunity to experience some competencies • Redundancy may hinder completion requirements

Figure 4.6 SWOT Analysis to help achieve a goal.

identified, and appropriate milestones considered, when it comes time to formally planning how these goals will be achieved, a further process of goal consideration is advisable. Once you have completed a SWOT, it is key to ask yourself, 'Now What?'. Whilst undertaking a SWOT is recommended, it will only take you so far. Building upon the elements identified is key. For example, now you have identified weaknesses, how can you address them? After you have developed the elements identified in the SWOT, goals and milestone can start to be set. To ensure all goals and milestones are as effective as they can be, it is good practice to ensure all goals and milestones are SMART.

4.7.2 SMART goals

SMART is an acronym that helps guide goal setting. Table 4.3 explores the SMART acronym in greater detail with an explanation of each element and

Table 4.3 SMART goals

S	Specific	It is important to ensure all goals and milestones are specific so no ambiguity exists. Questions that can be considered include what is the goal I want to achieve? Who is involved in the goal? The more specific a goal is, the easier it will be to visualise, understand, and ultimately achieve.
M	Measureable	The progress of any goal must be measured. By knowing progress has been made, you are closer to achieving the goal, motivation can be maintained, and the goals and milestones feel more manageable and achievable. Questions that can be asked to ensure a goal is measurable include can progress against this goal be measured? How will I know if I am on target to achieve the goal? Are there any metrics that can be used to monitor and assess progress?
A	Achievable	All goals set must be realistic and achievable. This is not to say goals cannot show a high level of aspiration. But impossible goals are by their very nature going to be impossible to achieve. Questions that can be asked include how will this goal be achieved? Is it realistic given the other parameters such as the time in which it is required to be complete or with the resources that are available?
R	Relevant	The goals with the highest likelihood of successful achievement are the ones that are relevant to the individual seeking to achieve them. The reasons may be personal or professional, secret or widely discussed. Questions that may help determine a goal's relevance include is the goal relevant to current and future career plans? And why do I want to achieve this goal?
T	Time bound	The key to the success of any goal is knowing exactly when it should be completed. First, it allows us to immediately assess how realistic achievement is going to be and helps us manage our expectations accordingly. There is nothing wrong with being optimistic (this is encouraged in goal planning), but there needs to be enough time between when the goal is set and its deadline for it to be realistically achieved. Second, a deadline allows for milestones to be identified so effective planning of expected progress can be mapped. Questions that may help this step include when do I want to achieve this goal? How will I know when this goal is achieved? What are the important dates that influence this goal?

how it relates to a goal or milestone. Whilst SMART does not have to be followed, without ensuring all goals are SMART, they will range from being difficult to impossible to truly achieve. Achievement of a goal or milestone is when a certain criterion, outcome, or level has been reached. Ensuring goals are SMART helps us understand this criterion so we can ensure what is achieved is exactly as intended.

SWOT analysis can help us both think of goals and also help further understand what is required in achieving those goals. Ensuring all goals and milestones set are SMART will ultimately ensure they are achievable. However, there is also a prevailing idea on the use of FAST goals.

4.7.3 FAST goals

Whilst FAST goals may not be as well known as SMART, they have been around a while and take a different approach to goal setting (Table 4.4):

Table 4.4 FAST goals

F	Frequently discussed	Goals should be openly and constantly discussed. They should remain a topic of conversation between staff and embedded in regular monitoring sessions. Progress can then be subject to scrutiny and support with evaluation and feedback provided to help ensure the goals remain current and everyone is aware of their importance.
A	Ambitious	Any goal should be difficult to achieve but not impossible. Whilst some milestones may be easier and more straight forward to accomplish than others, care should be taken to strike the balance between ambitious goals that will push and develop skill sets and those goals that are simply impossible to achieve given any constraints that are in place, such as resources and time. However, it is always important to ensure optimism exists and ambitious goals are set.
S	Specific	An understanding of what is needed to achieve a goal is required. This can take the form of a set of milestones that serve as a programme for what will be achieved and by when. The more specific the milestones, the easier it will be to understand what is required to reach them, and the easier it will be to see the part they play in the overall achievement of the goal.
T	Transparent	The key to FAST goals is transparency. All goals set, milestones planned, and progress made are transparent for all colleagues to see. The 'public' nature serves to add an element of pressure to continue against each goal when set, as colleagues will be able to see all (or lack of) progress. It also allows for a more supportive, collaborative, and inspirational company culture. However, negative aspects also exist, such as the reluctance of some to share goals they consider personal and how a lack of progress due to a personal issue's others may not know about could be perceived.

The idea of FAST goals has been argued to originate from the concept 'management by objectives' that was first introduced by management consultant Peter Drucker in his 1954 book *The Practice of Management*.

Management by objectives is the sharing of goals between employee and employer, with the openly available goals arrived at ideally in a collaborative manner but with an employer-focused benefit. The employee can then see their own progress against each objective they achieve increasing the sense of purpose and accomplishment they feel. Although the approach is open to abuse by employers who potentially mismanage the process by taking control of the objective setting, use it as a method to embarrass those who do not progress as expected or foster a culture where achievement of objectives is focused on at all costs creating an overly competitive and anti-collaborative organisational culture. That being said, if employed correctly management by objectives can yield to a collaborative organisational culture between both employees, and also between employee and employer. This approach, and variations of it, has been utilised by many leading software and technology companies in the personal and professional development of employees.

There are arguments that the concept of FAST goals should be used instead of that of SMART goals (Sull and Sull, 2018). However, the two are not mutually exclusive. Whilst there is some overlap in certain aspects of each (notably the 'S' standing for 'specific' in each), the principles of both complement one another if combined correctly. SMART is arguably a personal tool for identifying goals that are of personal importance (either personal or professional goals) whilst FAST is a more 'public'-focused approach in that it is a process of shared goal setting and development between employee and employer. However, using elements from both can help identify more robust and focused goals for development.

4.7.4 STEEPLE analysis

STEEPLE analysis combines and builds upon analysis methods such as STEEP, PEST, and PESTLE. It is effectively a business analysis tool and so it focuses more towards identifying market factors for organisational decisions. When goal setting, however, it is prudent to be aware of, and utilise, all the potential tools that may offer some assistance. This is where a STEEPLE analysis comes in. It helps with the focus of ideas and the consideration of wider factors that may influence the success of an idea or concept. These lessons can be transferred to goal setting and help with the identification of factors and barriers to goals that may not be immediately identified or fully understood without further deliberation. STEEPLE may be ideally placed with some goals, as many goals that are set are the development and launch of new ideas, and so STEEPLE sits nicely with these in consideration of the 'macro' factors that may impact upon the goal's success. STEEPLE is elaborated upon further and linked to goal setting in Table 4.5.

Table 4.5 STEEPLE goals

S	Social	This relates to elements such as business culture as well as wider social trends in society. Where is society heading, and what are the types of organisations that are thriving and struggling? Consideration of wider elements can help in the identification and setting of goals. The development of new technology will always bring change.
T	Technological	For goal setting this could be an awareness of the technology available to you, the technology you will need, or the changes you forecast arriving due to developments in future technology.
E	Economical	Wider economic factors should be considered in the planning of some goals. For example, if economic times are far from ideal, perhaps now it is not the best time to plan for immediate pay increases or push for expensive external training. But it could be an ideal time to shadow colleagues or initiate informal mentoring roles.
E	Environmental	Environmental concerns and movements could be a personal consideration based on your beliefs regarding climate change, and the actions you want to take to address this, whether as an individual or through your organisation. Such considerations could then become goals you set. Certain goals could also become more or less important in the eyes of those around you based on a changing environmental focus. Consideration of wider environmental aspects could help protect the focus on any goals you have.
P	Political	How does wider government policy and action influence your goal or idea? If your goal is to start or grow a business, you will ultimately be impacted upon by the government decisions of one or more country.
L	Legal	First, the legal element relates to being aware of, and abiding by, the appropriate and applicable legislation. It is obviously important to ensure all goals set are legal, and only legal means will be employed in their achievement. Second, an awareness of upcoming legal changes could provide opportunities for the setting of goals. If legislation is introduced that places increased responsibilities on certain parties (anything from procurement to health and safety), goals may need to be set to become up to date with the latest legal changes.
E	Ethical	Building on, but going beyond, the principles you may encounter in the legal considerations, ethics is more than if something is legal or not, and is concerned with if the decisions you make and the goals you set are ethical and the 'correct' things to do.

4.8 The setting of goals

The SWOT, SMART, FAST, and PESTLE analysis methods can aid with goal identification and setting techniques. They can be used in conjunction with one another, with each method complementing the others by allowing a further and more robust analysis of goal setting to occur. How these techniques 'fit' into the creating, developing, and setting of goals can be seen in Figure 4.7. If goals are set

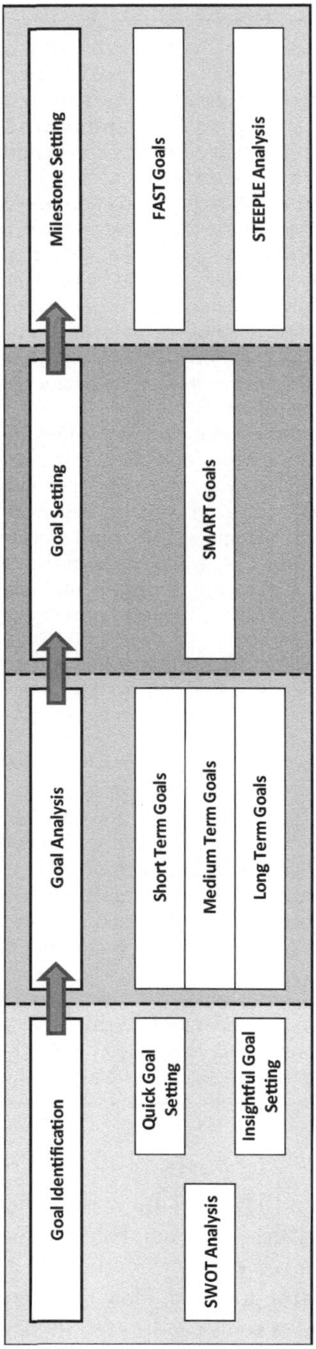

Figure 4.7 Goal Setting Model.

that are robust and the result of a well-thought-out process and deep consideration, they are going to be easier to visualise and plan with greater accuracy, and there the steps to achieve will be more focused and easier to follow, which will ultimately result in the goals being more likely to be achieved.

4.9 Conclusion

This chapter is concerned with the setting of goals. The idea of goal setting may appear straight forward as you may already be aware of the goals you want to achieve. However, if you are not aware of the goals you want to achieve or would like to consider wider goals not immediately apparent or applicable, or even break down existing goals to make their achievement more likely, then the techniques and methods outlined in this chapter will prove beneficial. If you already know every goal you want to achieve, then the techniques and methods outlined in this chapter will help you consider these goals in greater depth so they can be fully understood. Figure 4.5 shows how all these practices come together to help goal setting by offering a model for goal consideration, identification, reflection, and setting. In Chapter 5, these goals are built upon further with practices and techniques for the successful monitoring and completion of goals and milestones.

References

Drucker, P (1954). *The Practice of Management*. New York: Harper and Row.

Locke, E., Motowidlo, S. and Bobko, P. (1986). Using self-efficacy theory to resolve the conflict between goal-setting theory and expectancy theory in organizational behavior and industrial. Organizational psychology. *Journal of Social and Clinical Psychology*, 4, p. 328–338.

Sull, D. and Sull, C (2018). *With Goals, FAST Beats SMART*. MIT Sloan Management Review. Available from: https://sloanreview.mit.edu/article/with-goals-fast-beats-smart/

5 Goal planning

5.1 Introduction

This Chapter builds upon the foundation of how to set goals that was explored in Chapter 4. Once goals are identified, this chapter assists in the planning of goals including how to map out the journey that the achievement of a goal will look like and how to understand the processes involved in the achievement of goals, and the tools available that ultimately enable successful goal achievement. This chapter also helps individuals who set and manage the goals of another, whether that be a colleague or someone they line manage. The topics covered in this chapter will help a manager understand how progress against goals should be mapped and how milestones can be effectively set and accomplished to enable overall goal achievement. The processes can also be used by organisations generally, to implement professional development plans for their workforce that are realistic and provide the appropriate amount of support and guidance to help their entire workforce successfully develop their skill sets. In summary, once a goal is set, this chapter outlines how a continuing professional development (CPD) plan can be created around it to ensure its successful achievement.

5.2 Where to start?

The tools and techniques portrayed in this chapter presume goals have been set. Chapter 4 provides guidance on how to successfully set goals that are appropriate and clear enough to be achieved as intended. Whilst it is always possible to achieve goals without following the guidance set out in this chapter and in Chapter 4, by adopting the tools and following the guidance provided, goal achievement and therefore professional development will become a much more robust and efficient process allowing the focusing of energy and efforts to areas that will provide the most immediate return in terms of progress towards the goals identified. Once a goal has been considered correctly, it is time to include it on a CPD plan. The next stage is therefore to ensure the CPD plan is fit for purpose and developed around the goals set so the goals can be effectively and efficiently achieved. There are many techniques and practices that can be adopted when developing CPD plans and many concepts to be aware of. Although I suppose, as goals have already been identified in Chapter 4, some may ask the question: why do they now need to develop a CPD plan?

5.3 Why plan?

Planning for any task in life allows a sense of perspective to be gained. Such perspective includes if the task is achievable by the preferred date and what resources may be needed to assist in the task's completion. Planning also allows for a deeper comprehension of the commitment required to complete the task and identification of any difficulties that may be experienced along the way. Goal setting has been described as a successful technique to enable behaviour change towards effective goal achievement (Epton et al., 2017). However, despite the benefits of identifying goals, studies have shown that simply listing out goals alone rarely results in their achievement if the cognitive processing involved is minimal and goal commitment does not occur (Koestner et al., 2002). This can potentially be overcome with the techniques described in Chapter 4 of how to effectively evaluate and dissect a goal so a better understanding of it can be reached and the goal itself can become more refined and focused. Planning the achievement of a goal, however, such as required in a CPD plan, is the next step in helping the successful achievement of any goals identified.

The title of the 2020 paper by Michaela Schippers et al. published in the academic journal *Contemporary Educational Psychology* sums it up quite well: 'Writing about personal goals and plans regardless of goal type boasts academic performance'. In the paper, Schippers analyses the performance of four first-year undergraduate cohorts of students from a Business Administration degree course in the Netherlands. Two cohorts undertook the goal-setting exercises and two did not, and then their performance at the end of the academic year was compared. The cohorts who undertook the goal-setting exercises were found to have performed better academically. The results concluded that "in terms of practical significance, a personal goal-setting intervention is a relatively straightforward way to improve first year university student performance" (Schippers et al., 2020, p9). The results, however, transcend simple academic achievement and encompass general high performance in the attempt to achieve any goal set, especially as part of a CPD plan. The technique, according to the paper's findings, is to reflect on the goals set, strategise the attainment of these goals, reflect in writing about anticipated obstacles, and then develop plans aimed at specifically overcoming these obstacles. The results also revealed that higher performance in one area does not necessarily depend upon a task-specific goal being identified, i.e. the general process of setting goals and planning their achievement will help an individual's wider performance. It is therefore highly recommended that once a goal is correctly analysed and set, a plan is developed around the achievement of this goal. As most people will have multiple goals ongoing simultaneously (a mixture of short-, medium-, and long-term), the recording of these goals will become a CPD plan.

A CPD plan can then be used 'externally' as evidence to parties who need to see an individual's professional development objectives and be updated on any progress made towards these goals. For example, many of the professional bodies identified in Chapter 3 will require a candidate to keep and submit a CPD plan to be assessed as part of the requirements to join the professional body. Such professional bodies will then also require members to keep an ongoing CPD plan to evidence their continuous development. Line managers may also want to see colleagues' CPD plans as part of staff performance reviews that could be linked to promotions and pay increases. CPD plans can also be used 'internally' by the individual who created the plan as a self-assessment of the progress made against any goals set and can be used as a motivational instrument when goals may not be achieved as quickly as first anticipated.

Planning out the achievement of goals in a more methodological approach is therefore the next logical and practical step in achieving the goals, once they have been correctly identified and analysed. Planning has been described as central to self-regulation and helps reveal what activities are needed to be completed, when they need to be completed by, and how they can be completed. Indeed, it has been stated that goal planning "*acts like a map to move between actual state and goal state*" and that without such a CPD plan in place "*self-directed and goal directed activity is haphazard or at best a process of trial and error*" (Robinson et al., 2015, p32). Whilst the process of CPD planning may be guided by an employer, a professional body, or an individual themselves, the key underlying consistency needed for a successful CPD plan is for an individual to take responsibility for their own professional development, as well as the creation and updating of their own plan.

5.4 Taking responsibility

It is always good practice to be reminded that professional development, whilst benefitting to a company, is ultimately a personal responsibility. Some companies may place high emphasis and focus on the professional development of their employees, which will be of great benefit to both the employees and the company itself. Other companies may place no emphasis or importance on the professional development of their staff. In either example, the onus of professional development should always be upon the individual. A company which is proactive in staff development may not continue like this forever, or staff may find their development opportunities limited to those who directly help the company and are not easily transferable to other employers (i.e. training on a very company-specific piece of software). Therefore, employees should always maintain their own CPD plans with their own professional goals, even if just to ensure a company's development plans align with their own.

Similarly, staff who work for companies that do not encourage their employees to professionally develop (or worse, restrict, and hinder the development of employees) should also take responsibility for their own professional development. They should not wait for a company to begin a long-promised development programme before crafting their own CPD plan, and they should proactively identify their own goals and plan for their achievement. This is not to say staff should leave employers who do not focus on professional development. Just that in instances such as these, professional development opportunities should be sought from elsewhere. Research on the prevalence and motivations for construction companies supporting employees CPD conducted by Hurst (2009) revealed that staff development was driven by organisations seeking to mitigate skill deficiencies amongst its employees to maximise organisational performance. The same research also revealed that some organisations were hesitant to develop staff 'too much' for fear of them being 'poached' by competitors.

Working for an employer that provides many professional development opportunities and working for an employer that provides none ultimately leaves an employee with the same decision, out of all the professional development opportunities available, either internally to the company or externally, where should time and effort be focused to ensure maximum efficiency and CPD goals can be achieved in a timely manner, and energy and effort is not wasted on misdirected activities.

5.5 Return-on-time invested

Return-on-time invested (ROTI) is simply calculating if the 'return' gained from something is worth the 'time' invested to achieve it. A simple analogy is if a Project Manager (PM) needs to know whether the materials ordered for site will be delivered on the expected day. The PM could drive to the supplier's office and ask in person when the materials will be delivered, or the PM could simply phone up the supplier and ask. Whilst this example is simple and somewhat obvious, the same consideration should be given to all tasks professionals undertake, especially when concerning CPD.

Some goals will always take longer to complete than others. For example, you may need to gain a certain number of years' experience or there may be many hurdles to clear that will inevitably take longer to achieve than other goals identified. However, when it comes to professional development, it is prudent to ensure time is not wasted. This is especially important if time is wasted completing activities that were never required for the achievement of a goal in the first place, either through a lack of understanding of the requirements of a goal or by following a sub-optimal route to success. Effective professional development requires an effective ROTI. Whilst CPD targets will ultimately be achieved even without consideration of ROTI, the number of goals accomplished will always be lower, and the time taken to accomplish them will always be longer than they could have been had the idea of ROTI been considered in the development and undertaking of CPD plans.

5.6 How to break down goals

Once a goal has been identified and analysed, it should then be broken down into a series of actionable steps. Each step should also then follow the same structure of the overall goal (i.e. be Specific, Measurable, Achievable, Relevant and Time bound – SMART), and it should be easy to establish when each step has been achieved. For the purposes of this textbook, each step is then referred to as a milestone. Achievement of each milestone set will then serve as reinforcement and reassurance that progress is being made towards the achievement of the overall goal.

There are many methods of breaking down goals into subsequent milestones. One method, for example, could be based on the chronological order in which activities are required to be carried out. This is a relatively straightforward method as once the required order of completion is identified; these activities then naturally form each milestone. Another method could be the breaking down of a larger goal into all its constituent parts, and then identifying which of these parts can be achieved by the easiest means, before putting these as the first milestones to complete. This will allow relatively quick progress to be made along the first few milestones and could potentially help build enthusiasm and motivation to complete the rest. Alternatively, the hardest milestones could be attempted first so that it is 'downhill' from that point onwards. Another method of breaking down a larger goal into a set of subsequent milestones could be a time-efficient one, which allows focus on each different milestone at a time that suitably aligns with different commitments or existing goals and milestones.

In most cases, the method of breaking a goal down will be somewhat obvious initially, in that once a goal is analysed, milestones to its success will become apparent. However, in such circumstances, it is only by deeper analysis and consideration of the goal that the milestones can be truly understood and planned effectively. Examples of milestones and goals can be seen in Table 5.1:

Whilst the above milestones could also be broken down further, they are included in Table 5.1 to act as an illustration of the broad steps that goals could be

Table 5.1 Example of milestones

Milestone 1	*Milestone 2*	*Milestone 3*	*Milestone 4*	*Goal*
Research professional bodies, select and apply for membership	Understand full requirements and timeline required	Complete entry requirements – i.e. diary completion and CPD log	Prepare for final submission of documents	Become Chartered
Research job profile for Senior Engineer	List all skills required currently not possessed	Identify training on skills required	Hold regular meetings with line manager	Promoted to Senior Engineer
Identify universities where qualification is offered	Complete business case for line manager	Ensure time is set aside to complete	Arrange mentor with previous MBA experience	Achieve MBA
Review previous tender documents sent to clients	Identify potential new clients and client requirements	Shadow bid team on new tender documents	Be part of bid team and contribute to submissions	Win work from new clients

broken down into. Once goals are also identified as short-, medium-, and long-term, some goals may then become milestones in the achievement of others. For example, Table 5.1 could become an individual's short-term CPD plan, with their long-term CPD plan represented in Table 5.2.

Table 5.2 Long-term milestones

Milestone 1	*Milestone 2*	*Milestone 3*	*Milestone 4*	*Goal*
Become Chartered	Promoted to Senior Engineer	Achieve MBA	Win work from new clients	Start own consultancy

It has been argued that the milestones of long-term goals can be translated into a set of short-term goals, and then the achievement of each of these short-term goals serves as reinforcement and evidence progression is being made towards the overall long-term goal (Robinson et al., 2015). This is reinforced in the book *Progress Principle* that analyses diary entrants of 238 people and argues that the most successful people are focused upon achieving 'small wins' (Amabile and Kramer, 2011). However, if it is difficult to break down any goals, or even know where to start in achieving any milestone, tools such as 'brainstorming' or 'mind mapping' can help. These are simple exercises that can be done alone or in groups, whereby a problem (in this case the achievement of a goal) is set and any ideas or potential solutions are named, wrote down, and then reviewed. This can help 'join up' two or more perhaps previously unrelated areas or see goals in more detail and a new light, and if the exercises are completed with others, their perspective can be gained which can identify and address things one individual alone may overlook. Whilst software is available to help these techniques and similar be adopted, and help with the analysis and discovery of patterns, the exercises can simply be completed with a piece of paper and pen. The key, however, when breaking down goals for inclusion in a CPD plan, is achieving the 'correct' balance between including enough detail on the goal and having a CPD plan that is simple and straightforward enough to be an easily amended document. CPD plans ultimately need to be evolving documents that are constantly reviewed, updated, and amended. They should not be only looked at once a year and then 'put in a drawer' until the next 'performance review'.

5.7 Balancing simplicity and detail

The level of detail CPD plans contain will ultimately be a highly personal decision. Enough detail is needed so that any goal can be clearly understood, and this is especially important if the plan is a public one, or one shared with colleagues or management. However, too much detail will result in a 'clunky' plan that is difficult to update, time consuming to review, and challenging to follow, all factors that could result in the CPD plan not being used as effectively as it could and therefore demotivating individuals and also potentially hindering the achievement of any goals identified.

In a study on the goals and objectives set as part of resource management planning, it was found that poorly defined goals, considered without clear time frames, and without the ability to measure and track progress in a meaningful way, would contribute to goals not meeting the required criteria and becoming less likely to be achieved (Dominguez-Tejo and Metternicht, 2018). However, having a goal to achieve in the first place can create an internal 'tension' between an individual's actual current state and their 'goal state', and to resolve this tension requires action to be taken (Robinson et al., 2015). The goal creating this tension, if not explored and analysed thoroughly, can lead to a haphazard CPD plan where the process of achieving a goal and any subsequent milestones can become obscure. It is therefore important to adopt the use of tools such as SWOT (Strengths, Weaknesses, Opportunities, Threats) analysis when considering the goals and also to ensure all goals *and* milestones are SMART. This will aid with clarity and focus and go some way to resolving this tension as there will be a clear and achievable path to the 'goal state'.

5.8 Creating a usable CPD plan

It may at this point appear to some to be counter-intuitive, in that you have identified a goal or series of goals that you want to achieve, and yet instead of 'seizing the moment' and heading straight off to achieve the goal, this book is advising further deliberation and consideration, which may appear to be holding back progress in goal achievement. However, to ensure an efficient ROTI is achieved, it is vitally important that effort is focused on the areas it will make the largest difference. Such areas are only identified with a little more time and effort spent at the start of the process clearly mapping out how the goal can and should be achieved. Time spent creating a CPD plan before goals and milestones are attempted to be achieved will save much more time later in the actual undertaking of the milestones on the way to achieving the goals set.

The first step in creating a useable CPD plan is to search for existing templates. This may be easy if a template is provided by an employer, but if not, a quick online search will reveal many examples that can be downloaded free of charge. If an online template is found that suits an individual's need and layout preferences, then it can be used and will suit that individual's development plan perfectly, but this will be quite rare as the majority of CPD plan templates do not include all the categories, headings, and sections that will ensure they are truly fit for purpose and serve as an effective mechanism in helping achieve any goals set. If a template is found that does contain some elements that are useful, this could then be amended by an individual to suit their own development needs.

Section 5.11 contains examples of CPD plans, but those contained act merely as examples of templates that could be built upon to suit individual needs. CPD plans could also be created from scratch. Faced with a blank piece of paper could

Table 5.3 Common elements to include in CPD plans

Element to include in CPD plan	*Description*
Clearly defined end goals	A detailed analysis of the goals set will need to be undertaken so any goals can be fully understood. All goals should be SMART.
Appropriate milestones	Once a goal is broken down into manageable steps, these will then become the milestones, with each milestone being SMART and identified for completion in a logical manner.
Realistic reflection of current position	It is only by having a honest understanding of their current position, ability, and limitations will an individual be able to improve their skill sets and so maximise the potential a CPD plan offers.
Ability to update and amend all details easily	The ability to make changes easily when they are encountered, whether goals have been accomplished and need to be removed, or milestones are changed as more information becomes available, is essential for a CPD plan to remain up to date and relevant.
Clear and easy to follow format	This will be of benefit if the CPD is personal or shared, as an easy-to-follow format leaves little room for confusion about what is the next milestone that needs to be completed.
Mixture of professional and personal goals	Whilst CPD plans can be entirely personal or professional, a mixture of both types of goals (or two separate plans) can be highly motivational. As there is also a blurred line between the boundaries of both types of goals for some people, having an exclusively personal or professional CPD plan may not reflect current lifestyles.
Ability to monitor and update any progress made	As some CPD plans are shared with colleagues or line managers, the ability to evidence progress made against goals is key. Even if the CPD plan is personal it can increase motivation and satisfaction to see progress be recorded against each goal set.

be daunting for some but offer freedom for others and allow a unique and truly bespoke CPD plan to be created. The key lesson to the creation and use of any CPD plan is a document that works for the user. It must be clear and logical for the user to follow and update and also support the user in achieving their goals in the most effective manner. However, Table 5.3 contains some common factors that would benefit from being considered for inclusion in all CPD plans.

5.9 Monitoring and recording progress

In a study looking at how professional development can be embedded in student and graduate behaviours, Maddocks and Sher (1999) encouraged participants to proactively develop skills and record all achievements in a RAPID (Recording Achievement for Professional and Individual Development) Progress File. This

Table 5.4 Different methods of measuring progress

Method of measuring progress	*Description*
Percentages (%'s)	This could take the form of a percentage next to each milestone. These can then be updated whenever progress is made, or at set review times (i.e. monthly). Whilst %'s are subjective, as what is a 5% increase to one person may differ to the next, CPD plans are personal. Therefore, the subjectivity may not be a large issue, and instead serve as a motivating factor to see the %'s increase and the overall goal achievement become closer with each update.
Colour coding	Goals or milestones could be colour coded to show general progress made. For example, milestones could be green if achieved or on target, amber if actions are currently being taken, and red if behind schedule. The benefit of this method is that it easily identifies which goals and milestone need urgent action to prevent them from failing and becoming unachievable (i.e. if something is time bound).
Tick boxes	Having boxes next to each milestone that are then ticked when that milestone is complete is clear and easy to follow, and it is easy to share with others any progress that is made. However, this relatively simple method does not illustrate any progress made that does not result in the completion of a milestone.
Bar charts	Bar charts are a very visual representation of progress towards some goals, especially when such goals and milestones can be easily quantified. Bar charts can also be overlapped in different colours revealing changes in progress since the last review.
Progress lines	Lines that are extended to show progress are again a great visual representation of goal and milestone achievements. They can be edited and amended easily, and can also be used as an effective method of forecasting progress and form part of a joint progress review where an individual may indicate their own level of progress, and then a line manager indicates their understanding of the individuals progress level, with the lines acting as an easy-to-follow visual record.
Graphs	There are numerous graphs at the disposable of people with minimal computer skills, thanks to Microsoft Excel and other online graph generation software. Graphs in general are an effective way to display information, but for a CPD plan will require constant updating with each review to ensure they accurately reflect current progress. The selection of graph will have to be considered and will be dependent upon the goal set, the number of milestones, and the benefit a graph will bring. Having something visually attractive but that serves no real purpose will increase the amount of time updating the CPD requires and so may have an adverse effect of decreasing motivation and enthusiasm for updating the CPD regularly.
Removal of old milestones once complete	One method of measuring progress could be to simply remove old milestones once complete. The benefit of this is that it will allow a CPD plan to keep as much current and relevant information as possible without the plan becoming unmanageable and taking up too many pages. However, the disadvantage of this is that any progress may be forgotten if it is not visible on the plan which could lead to demotivation and will also become more difficult to easily illustrate progress made to others, such as line managers.

is similar in aims and nature to the CPD plans outlined in this textbook. The study found that many participants expressed difficulties in reflecting upon their own competency levels, gathering evidence to support their competency assessments, and creating an 'action plan' for skills development (Maddocks and Sher, 1999). It is therefore vital that goals and milestones are correctly considered and CPD plans allow for goals to be monitored with the ability to update and record progress. Therefore, all CPD plans should have an effective mechanism in place to enable the completion of any milestones and goals to be recorded. Witnessing any progress being achieved, as well as the satisfaction gained from moving closer to a goal, will ultimately support continued motivation. There are many methods and mechanisms that could be implemented when measuring the progress made against milestones and goals. Table 5.4 describes how some of these mechanisms could operate:

It is also important that review periods are built into the fabric of any CPD plan, so that a regular appraisal against any progress (or lack of) that is made can be identified and reflected upon for lessons learnt. Perhaps goals and milestones need to be considered in further detail, or even reconsidered entirely if plans change and other opportunities present themselves. The intervals at which CPD plans should be considered will vary depending upon the context in which they were created. For example, professionally focused CPD plans as a result of workplace requirements may only be considered by a line manager on an annual basis, whereas personal CPD plans may be considered on a weekly or monthly basis. There is no right or wrong solution; it is whatever is right for an individual and their context. A mixture of personal and professional goals, reviewed regularly, even if workplace procedures do not require it to be so, will ultimately lead to a more effective CPD plan and an increased likelihood of goal success. Figure 5.1 is a process map of a CPD review that could be followed by an individual when reviewing progression against their CPD plan.

5.10 To share or not to share?

The sharing of CPD plans is a contentious issue. For some, it is a personal journey, and so sharing goals, whether personal or professional, is not something they are comfortable with. This can also extend to the milestones along the way. There is nothing wrong with this, but at some point, some goals will need to be discussed with others, especially when others are involved in their achievement. There is no need to be ashamed of any goals; if they are important enough to set as a goal, then they are important enough not to be embarrassed about and to openly discuss. It can be difficult in some circumstances, especially in a work setting, to share personal goals, and even sharing some professional goals may be difficult with colleagues if they are concerning promotions, pay increases, and other potentially confidential information. There is also often a 'fear factor' involved in that if goals are shared openly, and they are not then achieved, or progress is delayed, an individual may feel they may be judged by others. This need not be the case, but as only the individual who is setting the goal knows how and why they want to achieve it, keeping some details undisclosed for a set period of time is perfectly acceptable.

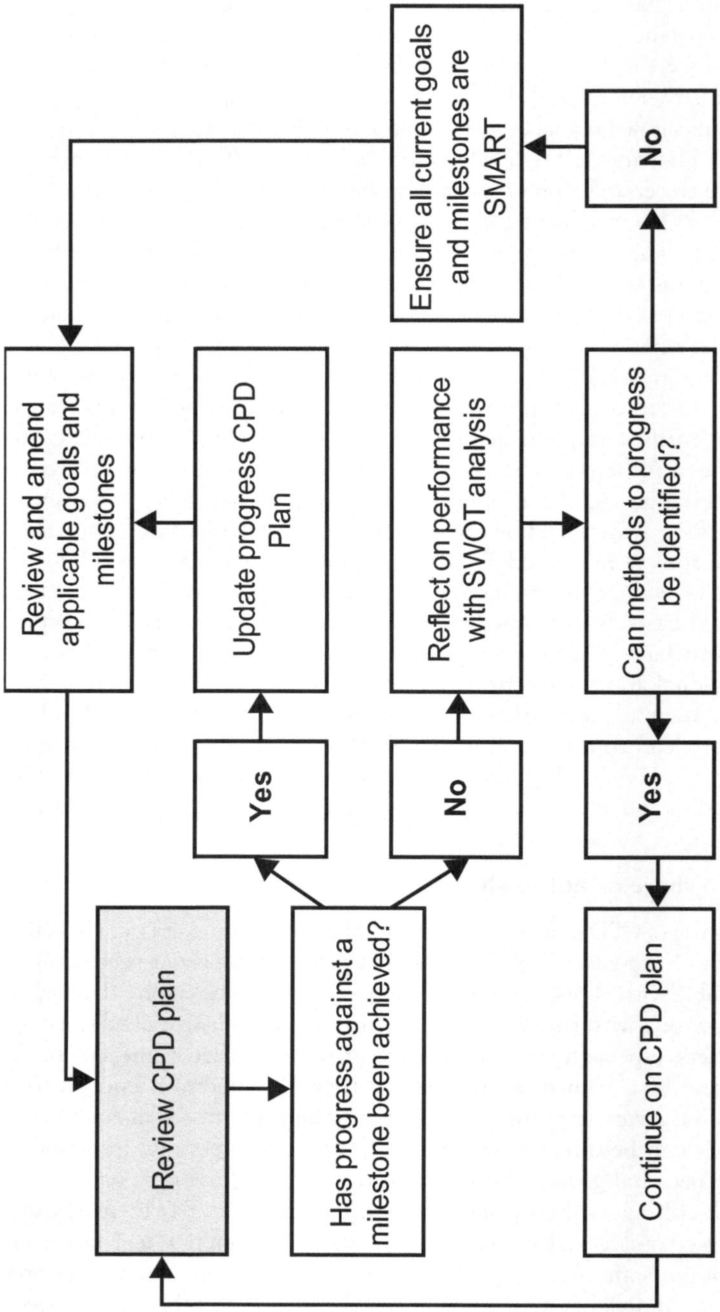

Figure 5.1 CPD review process map.

There are, however, many benefits to sharing goals with others, whether this is friends, family, strangers, or work colleagues and line managers. It has been argued that setting and the general achievement of goals is much more effective when it is public (Epton et al., 2017). Objective and Key Results (OKR), as discussed in Section 5.11, is essentially a shared goal-setting and progress updating method that utilises the support of colleagues as a motivational driver for individuals to achieve the goals set. Sharing goals via a variety of methods can also help ensure progress is made, as it will mean support is more forthcoming and an increased awareness of your goals and milestones will help others offer support and advise where possible. However, regardless of if a CPD plan is a purely private journey, a public pursuit, or somewhere in between, the form the CPD plan should take will need to be functional and effective.

5.11 Examples of CPD plans

OKR is a well-known personal and professional development goal-setting mechanism. It consists of an individual setting an objective (a goal) and then for this objective around five key results (milestones) are set. Both the objective and each of the key results need to be SMART with a particular focus on how each key result is to be measured. Once metrics are set, progress is then updated against these targets, and any progress made against each key result will automatically increase the overall progress made against the objective set.

Developed in the 1980s and favoured by technology companies, OKRs are often a ‘public’ manner of setting and achieving goals, with the OKRs of all employees made visible to one another within a single organisation. This has both advantages and disadvantages as discussed in Section 5.10. An example of how an OKR may look can be found in Figure 5.2.

Another simple method of goal performance measurement is to utilise KPIs (key performance indicators). A goal is set, with the success of that goal clearly defined (i.e. to run 26 miles in one go). Progress is then monitored and recorded with the indicator showing current achievement levels towards the total required, i.e. 15 out of 26 miles achieved to date. In an organisational setting, a KPI could be used to agree a required behavioural expectation or contractual requirement, for example the number of apprenticeship positions created by a main contractor

Objective:		**/100%**
Key Result 1:		/100%
Key Result 2:		/15nr
Key Result 3:		/32 visits
Key Result 4:		/100%
Key Result 5:		/60 emails

Figure 5.2 Objectives and Key Result.

during the construction of a project. This is a simple method of goal achievement and is used more at a high level to report progress, with the same analysis and detail required for the consideration of the goals and identification of all milestones.

There are also many unique and bespoke approaches to goal setting, milestone identification, and general CPD planning. Figures 5.3–5.7 illustrate the form some of these methods of CPD planning can take.

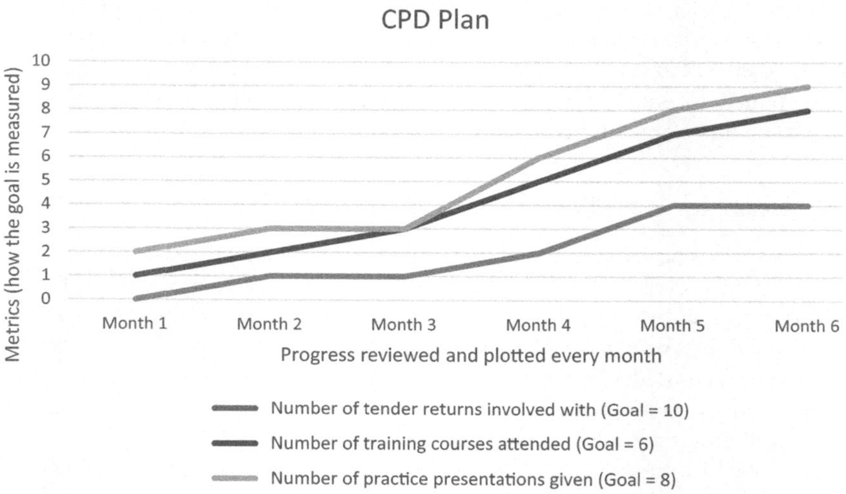

Figure 5.3 CPD plan Example 1.

Figure 5.3 is a method by which progress against a small set number of numerically measured goals can be monitored. In this instance the X axis is the review periods, so progress will be monitored, updated, and recorded each month. At this monthly review the number achieved to date against each goal would be updated, and the graph represents progress made. The Y axis can illustrate both the current progress of each goal and the forecast position. In Figure 5.3 three different goals are plotted, however one goal could be plotted using two lines. The first line would show the actual progress achieved to date against a set goal, and the second line could show the forecast or anticipated progress that needs to be made each month to ensure the goal remains achievable. When updated each month if the first line (actual progress achieved) is constantly lower than the second line (forecast progress made) then it will indicate actions are required to address the reasons why goal progress is not meeting early expectations.

In Figure 5.3 three goals are represented, one by each line plotted. This method of CPD planning is not ideal to keep track of multiple goals as the graph can become easily overwhelmed with multiple lines and be difficult to easily see if interim targets are being achieved. Also, using a method such as this may also make progress against some goals appear either more or less than has actually been achieved. A difficulty when using several lines on a single graph is they all may have different end goal amounts. If in the example provided the goal number of tender returns to be involved in was 100, this would make the goal line for tender returns appear much higher compared to the others, even though the other goals may be closer to be being complete.

Number	Goal Title	Date Goal Set	Date to achieve by	Details	Progress %	Date last updated	Reflection
1	Main Goal Title						
1.1	Milestone 1						
1.2	Milestone 2						
1.3	Milestone 3						
2	**Promoted to Associate**				**35%**		
2.1	Complete MSc	23/09/2020	04/07/2022	Ongoing PT - one night per week	**20%**	29/01/2021	Finding time to attend but need to find more time to complete work to higher standard
2.2	Finish project ABC	15/04/2020	14/04/2023	Currently PM - project value £65m	**35%**	29/01/2021	Project progressing as expected
2.3	Gain experience in department XYZ	01/01/2021	30/06/2021	Make contact with Emily for shadowing opportunities	**50%**	29/01/2021	Making good progress. Need to get dates agreed with all staff for time to shadow them.
3	Main Goal Title						
3.1	Milestone 1						
3.2	Milestone 2						
3.3	Milestone 3						

Figure 5.4 CPD plan Example 2.

The CPD plan in Figure 5.4 has taken the format of a table that outlines all key information relevant to the achievement of a goal. A quick inspection of the plan reveals that the goal set, in this instance, is 35% complete. The percentage complete of each milestone can also be viewed, and it is the average of these that automatically calculates as the total goal percentage complete. All goals set can be broken down into milestones and listed directly underneath each goal, these can be sequential or can simply be the core milestones that need to be achieved. Often milestones will run at the same time or have large overlaps in their completion. This method of CPD planning allows milestones to be easily listed and updated and can help increase motivation if the percentage complete increases (even if only slightly) with each update of the CPD plan.

This method of CPD planning also enables goals and milestones to be updated easily with changing details and circumstances. Milestones may change or grow, and this method accommodates such amendments easily. Percentages however, when used in self reflecting tools such as this, are subjective and so sharing progress made against one milestone may open the CPD plan up to scrutiny as someone else may believe the same progress is worth 10% more or 10% less than you have awarded. This should not act as discouragement to adopt a method such as this, as CPD plans are ultimately a subjective tool used to serve one primary purpose – to enhance the abilities of the CPD plan owner. If this method serves to do that, then regardless of scrutiny and arguments around subjectivity, elements of it should be adopted.

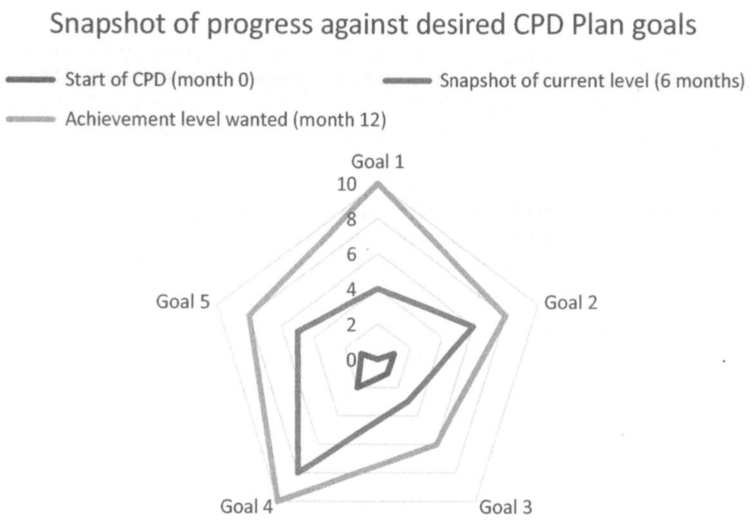

Figure 5.5 CPD plan Example 3.

The CPD plan in Figure 5.5 is another visual illustration of how progress against goals can be achieved. The same graphic could be adopted to illustrate the progress against several milestones all for one goal, or could, like in this example, but utilised for a 'high level' approach of just showing the progress against goals themselves. Whilst detail is lacking, this option could serve as a good summary of progress made towards goals, and if all goals have the same numerical metric target (in this instance lets say 10) then you know the close the loop gets to the outside of the graph to closer you are to achieving all your goals. Figure 5.5 shows three loops. The first, inner loop represents the ability level against each goal the CPD plan owner had when they started the process. The outer loop represents the ability level the CPD plan owner wants to achieve by a set date (in this instance 12 months after the plan was created). The middle loop is the loop that is updated with each review. The larger the middle loop gets (i,e. the more it moves away from the inner loop illustrating starting ability, and the closer it gets to the outer loop representing desired achievement level) then the closer the individual is to having achieved their goals.

No	Timescale	Goal	Success Criteria	Milestones	Obstacles	Motivation	Barriers	Start	Achieve by	Currently on target	Milestone Progress	Goal Progress

Figure 5.6 CPD plan Example 4.

Figure 5.6 is another table based CPD plan but has more options of analysis and detail included. It could be expanded upon further with specific reference made to the elements of SWOT and SMART included throughout. This allows for a much greater depth of analysis and goal exploration to occur, that really illustrates a substantial consideration for each goal. The more analysis that is conducted for each goal the more likely every important factor will be identified. The more information known about a goal, the more likely it is that the goal will be achieved. Having a thorough CPD plan will minimise the number of surprises that will be encountered on an individual's journey towards achieving any goal set. Being aware of the full requirements can allow accurate and realistic planning so expectations of all people involved can be managed accordingly (including the goal setter). However, the downside of such an approach can be it is a very time-consuming exercise to undertake, and too much information can make it difficult to update and illustrate clear progress. This can also cause problems when attempts are made to succinctly communicate elements of the CPD plan to others.

		Short Term		Medium Term		Long Term	
		Goal 1	Goal 2	Goal 3	Goal 4	Goal 5	Goal 6
Professional	Milestones						
	Opportunities						
	Threats						
		% Complete	% Complete	% Complete	% Complete	% Complete	% Complete
Personal	Milestones						
	Opportunities						
	Threats						
		% Complete	% Complete	% Complete	% Complete	% Complete	% Complete

Figure 5.7 CPD plan Example 5.

Figure 5.7 is a table format CPD plan, but this time with a different orientation of information. Columns and rows can be added, deleted, and amended as required, but this is a more sequential structure. Personal and professional goals can be separated and broken down into short, medium, and long term. How one connects to the other can be easily identified. For each milestone the immediate opportunities and threats can also be considered and included, ensuring that robust consideration is also given to each required step.

5.12 Conclusion

This chapter introduces the tools and practices of CPD plan development. It builds upon the setting of goals discussed in Chapter 4 and illustrates how these goals can be broken down into sequential milestones, and then how this information can be effectively plotted onto a CPD plan. Such a plan can then be reviewed and updated and any progress achieved can be recorded. This will help with maintaining motivation of goal achievement, and ultimately help achieve the goal itself, in the most time and resource efficient manner. Examples are provided of how

CPD plans could look, but such examples are provided for reference purposes only as the crafting of a CPD plan can be a highly personal pursuit with CPD plans bespoke and tailored, suiting individual needs and preferences when it comes to structuring goals and updating progress.

References

Amabile, T. and Kramer, S. (2011). *The Progress Principle. Using Small Wins to Ignite Joy, Engagement, and Creativity at Work.* Boston: Harvard Business School Press.

Dominguez-Tejo, E. and Metternicht, G. (2018). Poorly-designed goals and objectives in resource management plans: assessing their impact for an ecosystem-based approach to Marine spatial planning. *Marine Policy*, 88, p122–131.

Epton, T., Currie, S. and Armitage, C. (2017). Unique effects of setting goals on behaviour change. Systematic review and meta-analysis. *Journal of Consulting and Clinical Psychology*, 85(12), p1182–1198.

Hurst, A.G. (2009). CPD and work-based learning for construction managers: is it accessible? In: Dainty, A. (Ed) *Procs 25th Annual ARCOM Conference, 7–9 September 2009*, Nottingham: Association of Researchers in Construction Management, 523–531.

Koestner, R., Lekes, N., Powers, T. and Chicoine, E. (2002). Attaining personal goals: self-concordance plus implementation intentions equals success. *Journal of Personality and Social Psychology*, 83(1), p231–244.

Maddocks, A. and Sher, W. (1999). Introducing professional development at undergraduate level. In: Hughes, W (Ed.), 15th Annual ARCOM Conference, 15–17 September 1999, Liverpool: Liverpool John Moores University. Association of Researchers in Construction Management, Vol. 1, 33–41.

Robinson, O., Noftle, E., Guo, J., Asadi, S. and Zhang, X. (2015). Goals and plans for big five personality trait change in young adults. *Journal of Research in Personality*, 59, p31–43.

Schippers, M., Morisano, D., Locke, E., Scheepers, A., Latham, G. and de Jong, E. (2020). Writing about goals and plans regardless of goal types boosts academic performance. *Contemporary Educational Psychology*, 60, 101823

6 Reflecting on CPD

6.1 Introduction

Reflecting on continuing professional development (CPD) requires an understanding of what critical reflection is. For the professional or aspiring professional, understanding what a reflective practitioner is and how to become a reflective practitioner is crucial in personal development. This chapter looks at the concept of critical reflections and how it forms part of work-based learning (WBL) and practice-based professional learning (PBPL). To help in any personal development strategies, several reflective models have been explained with examples in use to support the reader's understanding.

Members of professional bodies are required to undertake CPD activities as part of the membership requirements. In respect of CPD activity, reflective practice is often used in two ways: first to determine which CPD undertakings will best support the required needs and second for post CPD attendance reflections on the effectiveness of the event.

6.2 Critical reflections

Reflecting on an experience or on an observed activity is an internal action and allows for a deeper understanding of that experience. You can reflect on an experience and in the process review your role and actions, perhaps draw a different conclusion so if you were to do the same activity in the future, you may do it differently. Implicit learning becomes part of this internal action.

For the modern professional, the act of reflecting forms a basis of learning and part of a continuous process for achieving growth or at least ought to be a continuous process and should not be limited to a one-time activity.

There are many professions that require a more reflective approach such as teachers and modern managers, for example construction project managers and those in senior management roles. These managers operate at a level that often requires hard and costly decisions to be made that will impact upon the firm's bottom line, the wider environment, and people's livelihood. Such managers will recognise the need for reflective practice and consequently will evaluate their own personal experience, identify strengths qualities and limitations, and take responsibility for their own continuous professional development where gaps in skills and knowledge become evident.

Reflecting is not limited to senior-level practitioners; for Higher Education and Further Education (the student), learners learning technical and vocational skills often lack the tools for critical reflection. Strategies such as WBL or work-centred learning and PBPL environments provide learners with the means to put into practice skills learnt and applied and allow for structured reflection to take place.

Critical reflection will add depth to an experience which is often articulated by a change in perception; although it does not always alter a future decision, it will, however, support the rationale behind the decision and provide a deeper understanding for such a decision.

There are many theories and definitions on 'critical reflection'. These often overlap with 'critical thinking', with both concepts frequently interchangeable in a professional setting. Both critical reflection and critical thinking are really aimed at solving problems in workplace environments. Critical thinking is aimed at looking for better ways of working or continuous improvement in the organisation, and critical self-reflection focuses on the individual in relation to their actions within the organisation. Both critical reflection and critical self-reflection are also frequently interchangeable.

In many industry sectors such as health care, critical reflective practitioners tend to operate in supportive organisations where time and profit constraints have a lesser impact and the need to improve care services is often the higher key performance indicator; these types of organisations encourage the practitioners to reflect. Conversely, employees working in competitive environments such as the construction industry are usually under pressures to finish the job on time and within budget and will have less time to think and reflect although post project reviews are an attempt to allow project participants a structured reflective opportunity to ascertain what went right and what didn't. Critical reflection can be a challenging part of professional life; and learning to be a critical reflective practitioner takes practice and will often require some form of training.

There are various models for critical reflection that can be used as an aid to reflect; the choice on which to apply is down to the individual and the working environment the individual operates within.

6.3 Work-based learning

For working professionals or those on modern apprenticeships at a college- or university-accredited vocational course, who typically would be studying part-time, or for full-time students on placements, WBL attempts to:

1. Connect what is learnt in the classroom to real live organisational situations
2. What is done in practice to the taught theory behind it

Being able to demonstrate learning while in a workplace environment can be considered WBL – from classroom to workplace. A workplace can be defined as

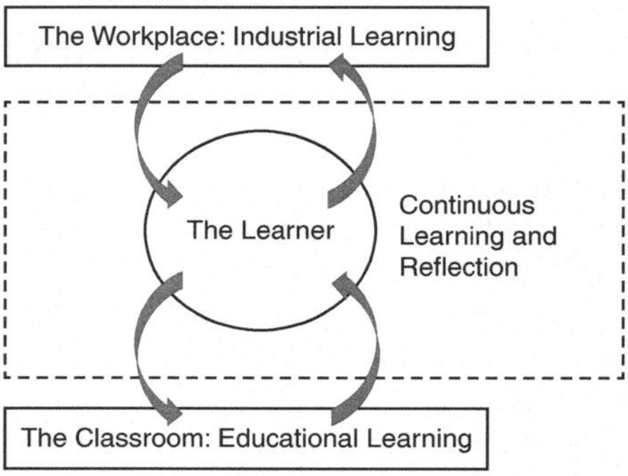

Figure 6.1 WBL model.

your permanent place of work or it can be simply a time-bounded activity such as work experience, placements, job shadowing, internship, and apprenticeships. The WBL model in Figure 6.1 demonstrates the relationship between learning and reflection and shows the learner at the centre reflecting in order to understand and enhance meaning between what is learnt in the classroom and what is applied in the workplace.

Many accredited on-site training courses can be included in this approach where structured assessments provide a means of demonstrating learning has taken place.

6.4 Practice-based professional learning

Similar to WBL, however, there is a distinction which is found in the 'professional' context and learning in practice. A professional in a practice through practice-based learning will develop the capacity to reflect and enhance their own knowledge through experience with the aim of self-and/or practice improvement. This model suggests a more lifelong learning approach rather than a single point of learning.

Examples of practice-based learning for professional disciplines can be found in the following professions:

- Medical
- Legal
- Architecture
- Accountancy
- Teaching
- Horticulture

To facilitate the development of skills through learning in practice requires an organisation to run as both a business and a learning practice usually in partnership with a university or other teaching organisation.

Approaches to PBPL include the following:

1 Structured activities (individual or collaborative) to learn and share good practice
2 Research solutions to enhance a more critical thinking approach
3 Reflect on practice to enable critical evaluation

In PBPL environments, some form of evaluation will take place and may need to be evidenced for professional bodies such as the Royal Institution of Chartered Surveyors through Assessment of Professional Competence (ACP) or the Royal Institute of British Architects' Professional Experience and Development Record.

Formal methods of assessing the learner may include an evaluation of technical, decision-making, leadership, and interpersonal skills, and can be in the form of written reflective portfolio. A mentor or assessor will assess this portfolio and decide if specific professional standards have been clearly demonstrated.

6.5 Reflective models

There are several theoretical models that can be adapted for WBL, work and PBPL all attempt to allow those in professional practices to become reflective practitioners for example:

1 Kolb's (1984) reflective model
2 Gibbs' (1988) reflective model
3 Schon's (1983) reflection-in-action/reflection-on-action model
4 Atkins and Murphy's (1993) model of reflection
5 Driscoll's (2007) model of reflection

Some are slightly more complex than others and are better suited to the type of learner and the profession.

6.5.1 Kolb's reflective model

David Allen Kolb was born in 1939 in Illinois, USA. He was Professor of Organizational Behaviour at Case Western Reserve University and Chairman of Experience Based Learning Systems (EBLS) and known for his research on experiential learning styles. Together with Ronald Eugene Fry, he developed the experiential learning model as published in his book *Toward an Applied Theory of Experiential Learning* (1974).

Kolb's reflective model also known as 'experiential learning theory (ELT)' provides a useful perspective to one's own learning and development. The four-stage experiential learning cycle in Figure 6.2 suggests that the learning process of an individual is essentially through discovery and experience. It is a circular process with distinct stages, this sequence of stages begins with a 'Concrete Experience'.

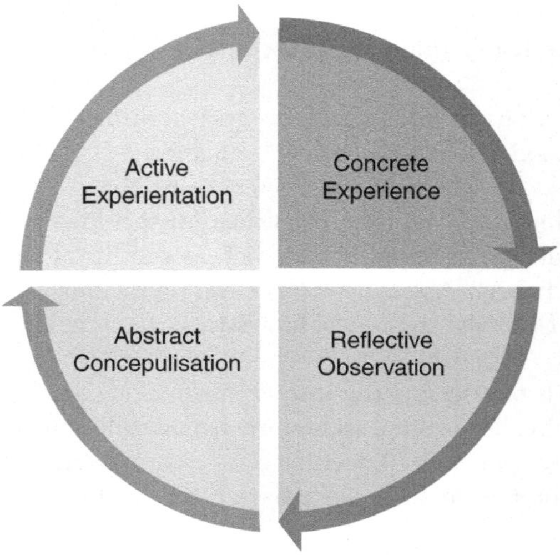

Figure 6.2 adapted from The Kolb ELT cycle.

Application by the learner.

1 Concrete experience (Do) – Describe the event/activity or situation.
2 Reflective observation (Observe) – Review the experience through some form of personal feedback.
3 Abstract conceptualisation (Think) – Develop new ideas in a systematic and structured way.
4 Active experimentation (Plan) – Apply new ideas and put into practice lessons learnt. This forms the basis of a new concrete experience.

The principles of the four-stage cycle are that the learner will follow the stages and acquire new knowledge and skills, and meaningful experience.

6.5.1.1 Example of Kolb's reflective model in action

You apply for the post of trainee site manager and have been asked to attend a formal interview at the head office of a large regional construction company.

Concrete experience – *You attend the interview and told you will be notified of the outcome by phone later that evening.*

Reflective observation – *Looking back, you feel overall it went well and you answered most but not all the questions you were asked. You came smartly dressed, but you thought you may have fidgeted too much. The interviewers seemed to like the amount of detail and content in your CV. But your knowledge of the company was limited and realise that you could have researched this much better.*

Abstract conceptualisation – *You begin to categorise all positives and negatives of the interview process. You answered most questions, you dressed correctly for the role, and you had a copy of your CV and application form at hand.*

Of the questions you did not articulate on, you now remember good examples, for example you could have mentioned some voluntary work you did that was not on you CV, and you could have done some better homework on the background of the company. You also recall aspects of interview training sessions you attended previously which have helped.

Active experimentation – *Although you weren't successful in getting the post, you know have an interview at a different company and plan to do more research on the company and think about transferable skills you learnt in your voluntary work such as team working in case you are asked for examples of teamworking.*

Although the four-stage learning cycle can be used to allow improvement by reflecting on an experience, Kolb recognises that not all learners learn the same way and what might be useful for one learner may not work for another, for example, at a broader level some prefer to be learnt or be taught in a structured traditional and formal way by watching and thinking, while others may prefer more interactive activities such as group work by doing and feeling. Kolb offers help to the learner by identifying four learning styles (Kolb, 1974), and it is knowing your preferred style in learning will help in reflective practice settings. These four styles are feeling, thinking, doing, and watching, and are paired as opposites on a continuum.

Feeling ---------- Thinking

Doing ---------- Watching

These pairs or opposites are directly linked to Kolb's ELT model in such a way (Figure 6.3).

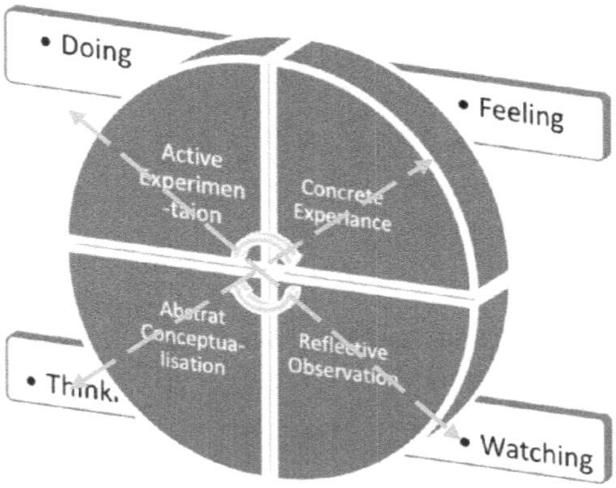

Figure 6.3 Learning styles adapted from Kolb (1974).

Table 6.1 Four learning styles

	Learning style	*Position in the learning cycle*	*Type of learner*
1	Diverging	Between the concrete experience (feeling) and the reflective observation (watching)	Open-minded Information gatherers Brainstormers Imaginative People person
2	Assimilating	Between the reflective observation (watching) and the abstract conceptualisation (thinking)	Logical Prefer ideas and concepts Practical Analysis situations
3	Converging	Between the abstract conceptualisation (thinking) and active experimentation (doing)	Problem-solvers Experimenters Technically minded Decision-makers
4	Accommodating	Between the active experimentation (doing) and the concrete experience (feeling)	Hands-on Intuitive Set targets Attracted to new challenges

Knowing your preferred learning style will help you to learn more effectively, Kolb's learning style inventory attempts to identify the learners preferred method, and thus, the learner will be better prepared focus on the learning activities that best suit the style; for example, a learner who identifies with a 'converging' or problem-solving learning style would be better suited to learn using practical-based activities (Table 6.1). The four advocated learning styles are as follows:

The types of learner traits are not set in stone and can overlap. The key is to make a choice of which one of the four best fits your own learning style, knowing it will help to learn more effectively.

Kolb's model is a widely accepted theoretical model, particularly in education. It is worth noting that the basis for applying Kolb's model is through experiential learning for most situations; in some limited instances, other theoretical models are better suited.

6.5.1.2 *Example of Kolb's learning styles in action*

According to Kolb, for effective learning to take place, learner must identify with one of the learning styles. Assuming learner has gone through the four learning styles and on balance opted for the 'Accommodating' learning style as their preferred choice, what is the course of action to be taken?

Answer

- Look for learning activities that sit within the learner's preferred style, for example on-the-job training, fieldwork, or simulation activities.

Conversely, attempting to apply the other styles can help to learn more effectively and broadly speaking activities that utilise all four learning styles through each of the four stages of the experiential learning cycle will fully support effective learning.

6.5.2 *Gibbs' reflective model*

In his book *Learning by Doing: a Guide to Teaching and Learning Methods*, Graham Gibbs (published in1988, Oxford Polytechnic, now Oxford Brooke University) identifies his reflective learning cycle theoretical model and shows how learners can apply it in their learning and teaching development.

Gibbs' reflective model provides an alternative way to learn from experience. Similar to Kolb's in its cyclical nature, the model identifies six stages for reflection and can be applied to single experiences as well as repeated events (Figure 6.4).

Application by the learner

1. Description – What happened? Explain the scenario, participants, roles, and expectations.
2. Feelings – Describe your feelings at the start and on reflection of the activity.
3. Evaluation –What went well and what did not? Yours and any other reactions to events. Use relevant theories to support your evaluation.
4. Analysis –Consider why things went well and why some aspects did not. Use relevant theories to support your analysis.
5. Conclusion – What have you learnt and what would you do or have done differently?
6. Action plan –Have you identified any gaps in your skills? How do you plan to fill the gap? Devise a revised strategy for the next time.

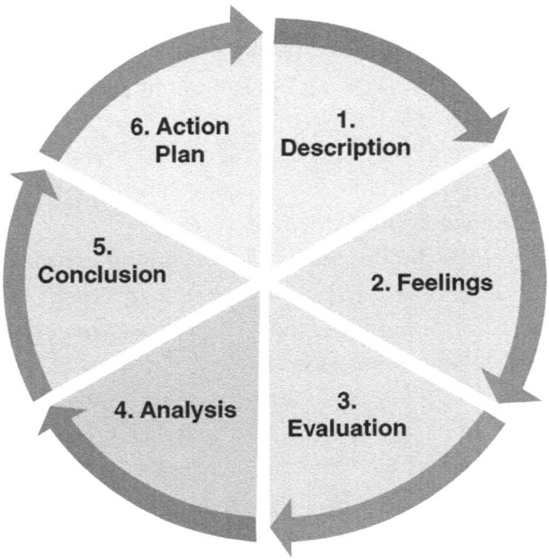

Figure 6.4 Reflective Cycle adapted from Gibbs (1988).

Gibbs' model is commonly used in the health care and education sectors but not limited to it. Some weaknesses of the model include difficulty by some users to describe and articulate their own feelings and this can be compounded in any further analysis when considering what went well or what did not go well.

6.5.2.1 *Example of Gibbs' reflective model in action*

A Quantity Surveyor is looking to broaden her skills into management and it has been agreed that she should attend a number of monthly site meetings with the main contractor in order to see how these meetings function and then chair a site meeting with the project suppliers to ascertain progress and confirmation of key delivery dates. The ability to chairing a meeting is a skill that will help her when applying for promotion in the future.

Following on from chairing the meeting, the Quantity Surveyor attempts to reflect on the experience using Gibbs' reflective model.

Step 1: Description – *Having attended several site meetings, it was my turn to prepare the agenda and chair a site meeting with suppliers.*

Step 2: Feelings – *Before the meeting I needed to prepare the agenda and make sure that those attending had agreed to the meeting date and would attend. I felt apprehensive because I thought they might reject my meeting requests due to their own workloads and not having 'senior' in my title. However, I got confirmations straight away which set my mind at ease. The agenda was less worrying as I had several agendas from previous meetings so just needed to change a few of the headings to suite the meeting. I made sure I had enough copies before the meeting. I did have a mild panic attack when I found out the site meeting room was already booked. But my manager intervened and freed up the meeting room for me. I tried to look as professional as I could throughout the meeting.*

Step 3: Evaluation – *The meeting overran by ten minutes, and the suppliers at times did not stick with some aspects of my agenda. I forgot to get teas and coffees booked for the meeting.*

Step 4: Analysis – *Looking back I could have kicked myself for not ordering the refreshments and should have taken better time control of the agenda and kept the suppliers focused on the agenda schedule.*

Step 5: Conclusion – *I am glad I chaired the meeting; the experience has helped my confidence, and I feel better prepared for the next meeting.*

Step 6: Action plan – *I have now created a checklist of things that need doing before a meeting to make sure I do not miss anything. I also need to pay strict adherence to the clock so as not to allow the meeting to overrun which can have a knock-on effect for my work colleagues. I will take my watch off and put it on the table to enable me to keep track of the time and will make the attendees aware of the importance of sticking to the agenda.*

The model to an extent is simple and superficial as there is little mention or suggestion to critical thinking. For those who have difficulty in exploring feelings, this model can be challenging to use. However, using the model helps to identify areas of strength and weaknesses and can also help to identify where skills require further development and training.

6.5.3 Schon's reflection-on-action and reflection-in-action model

Born in 1930 in Massachusetts, USA, Donald Schon pioneered the concept and development of learning systems. In his seminal book *The Reflective Practitioner: How Professionals Think in Action* (1983), Shon showed how professionals such as architects and engineers met the challenges of their work. This improvisation learned in practice for problem-solving was termed 'reflection in action'.

Unlike most of the other reflective models, the Schon's reflection-on-action and reflection-in-action model (see Figure 6.5) is not cyclical or stepped process. Schon suggests that two types of reflection takes place around a single situation, essentially a framework for thinking allowing for reflection to take place.

The concept of 'reflection in action' is to reflect on the activity as it is happening especially if the activity is going wrong and action is needed to rectify an ongoing problem. This is a reactive strategy, typically linked to prompt and urgent decision-making, where immediate solutions are often required.

The second type of reflection 'reflection on action' involves reflecting on the experience after the activity has ended. A more formal deliberate process that identifies what went wrong, why it went wrong, and how any lesson learnt can be used for the future. Table 6.2 identifies concepts associated with the timing of the reflection.

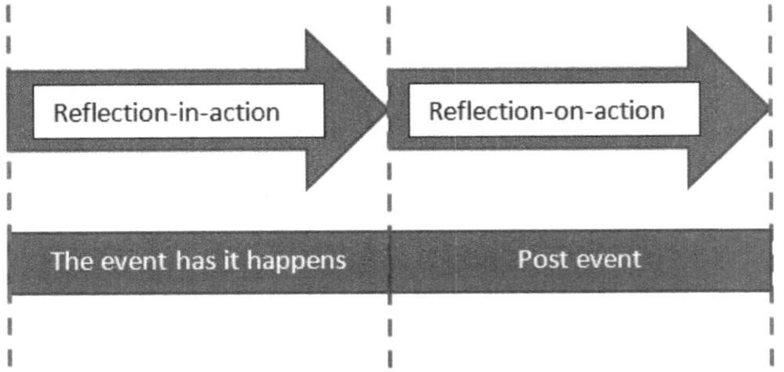

Figure 6.5 reflection-in-action/reflection-on-action model adapted from Schon (1930).

Table 6.2 Associated concepts of the timing of Shon's reflections

Reflection in action (in the event)	*Reflection on action (after the event)*
Reacting to a situation Experiencing Thinking about options	Looking back at the event What actions would you change? What went well?

Implementing 'how-to' reflective procedure models such as Kolb or Gibbs will support the Schon's model to assist the learner.

6.5.3.1 *Example of Schon's reflection-in-action model*

You are a manager working for a large regional roofing supplier supplying material to a large new build housing project that consists of the construction of 85 new dwelling, and as part of the contractor's team of suppliers, you have been asked to attend a site meeting with other suppliers in order to agree key dates of delivery and mitigate risks together with the site team.

Reflection in action

- *At the site meeting you find yourself distracted by a work order for another project and miss some key points from the meeting.*
- *In order to help stay focused, you quickly decide to switch you phone to silent and put it away in your briefcase and decide to make comprehensive meeting notes as you progress through the agenda items.*

Reflection on action

- *You realise that after similar meetings your recollections of actions are vague and can be potentially damaging to your company's bottom line.*
- *For subsequent meetings you ask in advance for an agenda for you to remind yourself of any key information requirements and write these under the correct agenda item.*
- *You also decide post meeting to liaise with the other suppliers to corroborate agenda actions and other key points.*

Schon provides a simple model of reflective practice by separating reflections whilst experiencing the activity and reflections in hindsight of the activity although it does not offer any detailed structured guidance for carrying out such reflections.

6.5.4 *Atkins and Murphy's model of reflection*

The Atkins and Murphy's model of reflection has its roots in the health care sector. Sue Atkins and Kathy Murphy developed the theory around the actions of stopping and thinking about the work activity and to explicitly analyse the experience to understand it and improve future actions.

The model (Figure 6.6) attempts to build upon the Gibbs' reflective model by supporting a deeper reflective approach. This model requires a learner to deal with emotions and deeper feelings, which can be for some an uncomfortable and personal experience. According to Atkins and Murphy, it is confronting these discomforts that personal development can be realised

Application by the learner

1 Awareness – Of discomfort or action/experience. Identify your emotions in relation to the event.

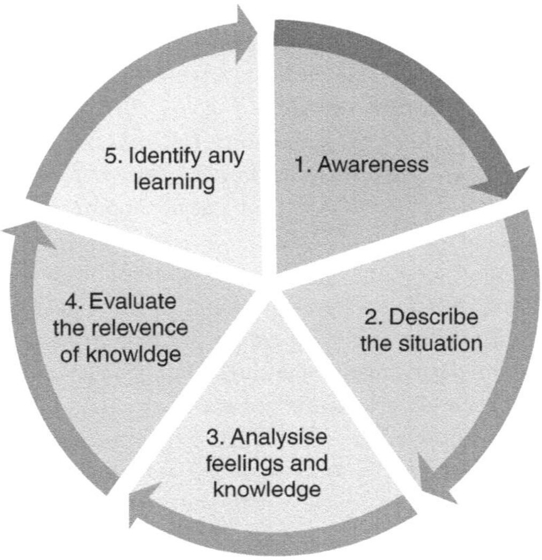

Figure 6.6 Adapted from Atkins and Murphy's reflective model (????).

2 Describe the situation – Include salient feelings, thoughts, events, or features. Identify your own involvement and those of others.
3 Analyse feelings and knowledge – Identify and challenge assumptions; imagine and explore alternatives. Were your assumptions correct/incorrect?
4 Evaluate the relevance of knowledge – Does it help to explain/resolve the problem? How was your use of knowledge? Build on the knowledge explored in step 3. Was the knowledge useful, and if not, why not?
5 Identify any learning – Which has occurred? Use the story you have built up in the previous stages to structure your reflections.

The Atkins and Murphy's model of reflection assumes that reflective learning occurs by facing discomfort; it requires the participant to be comfortable in making explicit these discomforts to be able to offer a critical analysis of the event. The skill to be self-critical requires honesty in any self-evaluation which may be difficult for beginners.

6.5.4.1 *Example of Atkins and Murphy's reflection-in-action model*

Awareness – *As a new trainee site manager, I was asked to support the assistant site manager at a site induction meeting for a number of new trades persons starting on–site, and a two of the trades were having difficulty understanding the assistant site manager as English wasn't their first language and the assistant site manager had a very broad regional accent. The event that transpired made me very uncomfortable, and my aim is to try and understand these feelings and use this understanding to help me deal with a similar event in the future.*

Describe the situation – *Four new plasterers were going through site inductions which included health and safety matters, Personal Protective Equipment (PPE), restricted areas, and work activities. Two of the plasterers used English as their second language, and it was evident to me having spoken with them that they were competent in communicating in English, if spoken to in a clear and deliberate tone.*

Throughout the one-hour site inductions, it looked like the two plasterers were taking notes and nodding as the induction progressed. When it came to my part of the induction, I told the new starters about the importance of wearing the right PPE and handed out gloves and glasses.

Later on that afternoon one of the plasters entered a sign-posted restricted area for an unknown reason and tripped into a trench badly injuring his arm. The site manager completed the necessary paperwork for an injury on site and gave me and the assistant site manager a threat of dismissal for incompetence. Later that evening I thought about the earlier events and became annoyed and upset about it all.

Analyse feelings and knowledge – *This a new job for me and my experience is very limited. I thought being asked to assist in the induction would give me valuable experience. My previous experience with site inductions was as an inductee I think I was out of my depth. The company rules on site inductions are clear and all new starters need to attend (S3 CDM 2015 regulations). Those new starter inductees did indicate to me that they understood the rules of the site, and although I did recognise the language barrier could be an issue, the assistant site manager leading on the induction did not. Communication is critical on site safety (Health and Safety Executive (HSE)) human factors briefing note on safety-critical communications). I was angry at the assistant site manager for not supporting me in the meeting with the site manager.*

Evaluate the relevance of knowledge – *Looking back at the event, it did provide me with some valuable lessons about communication and health and safety. So, the experience was useful. We were lucky the injury was not worse. In the induction we should have made sure the inductees fully understood the rule and obligations through better and more effective communication. At the later meeting with the manager, I should have explained my thoughts and not relied on the assistant site manager for support.*

Identify any learning –*Before any future induction, I need to make sure we fully communicate our requirements and recognise that local dialects can be problematic for this who use English as a second language. Our induction will include test questions at the end of delivery and before new starters are allowed on site.*

Atkins and Murphy's reflective model was specifically developed for health care workers such as nurses to reflect. Where there is human interaction and decision-making, it also has its place in other industry sectors.

6.5.5 Driscoll's model of reflection in action

John Driscoll first developed his reflective model in 'Reflective Practice for Practise' (1994) and can be found and built upon in his book *Practicing Clinical Supervision: A Reflective Approach to Healthcare* (2007). It builds upon the work of Terry Borton (1970) titled *Reach, Touch and Teach.*

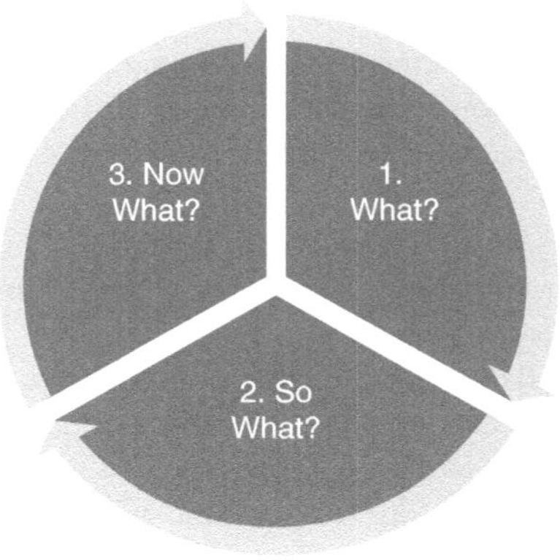

Figure 6.7 Adapted from Driscoll's (1994) model of reflection.

Driscoll's model of reflection is an effective method for reflecting on an experience and trying to learn from it. The main advantage of the model is that it is a simple and speedy process and gets us to consider three questions when reflecting on an experience. The three main elements of the model can be seen here (Figure 6.7):

Application by the learner

1 What? – Describe the event: what happened, what did you do, what did others do, how did you react?
2 So what? – Analyse the event: what did you feel, how do you feel now, what have you learnt?
3 Now what? – Propose actions following the event: what would you do differently, are you ready if it happens again? Action planning.

The purpose of Driscoll's model is to enhance your reflective practice skills. The aim of the 'what' is simply to set the context of the experience, and the 'so what' is the reflective elements and attempts to get you to articulate what has been learnt. The 'now what' or final stage is the application of lessons learnt if the same activity arises in the future. It is possible to conclude that you would do the same as before.

Due to its simplicity and speediness of application, it can lack a deeper reflective aspect.

6.5.5.1 Example of Driscoll's model of reflection in action

As a site manager I was asked by the head office to deliver a CPD event to the members of the site team. Knowing Driscoll's reflective model, I decided to use it to evaluate the event.

1 **What?** – *The CPD event took place on site in one of our temporary site cabins that were converted into a small classroom for inductions and meetings. Because*

I decided to combine this event with a team building exercise. The tables were set into four areas with three chairs to each table making four clusters. The plan was for the four groups to work on tasks and present their findings. Twelve members of staff attended the event which made four groups of three, and I prepared and delivered the session.

There was a 10-minute introduction to the topic, then 40 minutes working on the tasks, 40 minutes discussing the findings, and 10 minutes summarising the session.

2 **So what?** – *The challenge was for each group to prepare a site layout and traffic management plan based upon a given project scenario. This was a previous project I had worked on and I had a useful solution. Working in groups can be challenging, and I deliberately chose this way to show Tuckman's theory (1965) on team building in action and to show the groups how to recognise the issues and self-reflect on the challenge at the end of the session. The activity needed each group to communicate effectively on the task and on the presentation of the findings.* Lasswell *(1948) suggested a convenient way to describe what is communication is to answer the following questions: Who is the communicator? What is the message? What is the medium to be used to communicate? Who is the receiver? What will be the effect? The CPD event was for the attendees to consider the issues in designing optimum site layouts and safe traffic management systems.*

Each group identified different key factors in creating site layouts; most were unaware of the legal requirements. Peer learning was evident.

3 **Now what?** – *The event went well, and I would repeat the group cluster way of delivery next time. Some of the group members knew each other so communication and teamwork were largely frictionless, in the future I would swap the members around to make sure they didn't know each other, which would make it more challenging for them.*

Driscoll offers a quick way of analysing a situation and a chance to change things should the situation occur again.

There are many more models or frameworks for reflection, some of which are easier to understand and apply than others; for example, MacLean's (2016) weather model asks you to reflect on goals in practice using the analogy of four weather conditions:

- Sunshine as what went well
- Rain as what did not go well
- Lightning as what came as a shock
- Fog as what you did not understand

This model sets out a simple road map to allow the practitioner to reflect on an event or experience.

Rolfe et al.'s reflective model (2001) uses the same 'what', 'so what', and 'now what' questions as Driscoll but has a deeper aspect and the 'now what' element feeds straight back into the 'what' on a continuous loop.

No one model is the best one in all situations. A learner needs to choose one as a basis for reflecting and in the process can choose to change or alternate between some or create a useful hybrid. The key is to use a reflective framework that best fits a given situation. This is best achieved knowing and understanding various models in practice beforehand.

6.6 The reflective practitioner and CPD

This chapter so far has demonstrated how and why reflection is used and identified several structured reflective models that can help in reflective practice. Most models are similar and some more structured and detailed than others.

Fundamental to CPD is the recognition of the role of reflective practice; it is how you assess gaps in your skills, knowledge, or experience and understand fully the need to embark on further training. Reflective practice goes further than an aid to the identification of CPD needs it is also a post CPD tool that can confirm or otherwise if the CPD activity has met the needs gap.

CPD reviews are essential to the reflective practitioner's growth and development. It can also be a structured approach to ascertain the benefits of the CPD activity. A review should be undertaken in order to find the answers to questions such as:

- Did it meet my goal requirements?
- What can I take from the activity?
- Can I now use this in my professional development?
- Did it meet my needs gap so I can now perform better?
- Do I still need to do further activities?

These reflections form part of the reflective practitioner's CPD record as advocated by the industry's professional bodies. For those members of professional bodies such as the Royal Institution of Chartered Surveyors, the Chartered Institute of Builders, and the Institution of Civil Engineers. CPD is a regulatory requirement for the upkeep of professional competence and supports personal development. For those applying for membership, written evidence of reflective practice in action provides the critical element of the application process.

For annual staff appraisals or annual work reviews as required by many organisations, the answers provided by post CPD reflections will also demonstrate to the organisation how development goals have been met and are now being applied.

6.7 Conclusion

In WBL and PBPL environments, reflective practice is the principal mechanism that allows the professional to grow and develop. Reflective models support the professional in learning to be a reflective practitioner and at the same time offer a structured approach to personal development. Kolb's and Gibb's are the most well-known models; however, other models have been explored and the 'new' practitioner is free to select anyone or perhaps form a hybrid. What is essential is to have a structured approach to reflections, as it helps in the decision making on which CPD activities are based upon the practitioner's reflections and identified needs. Reflection does not end with the identification and fulfilment of the needs gap; it is also essential in post CPD reviews to answer the question: Has it met my development requirements?

References

Atkins S, Murphy K. Reflection: a review of the literature. Journal of Advanced Nursing 1993;18:1188–92.

Borton, T. (1970) Reach, Touch and Teach, London: Hutchinson

Driscoll J. (2007) Practicing Clinical Supervision: A Reflective Approach for Healthcare Professionals. Edinburgh: Bailliere Tindall Gibbs, G. (1988). *Learning by Doing: A Guide to Teaching and Learning Methods.* Free on-line at shop.brookes.ac.uk

Driscoll, J.J. (2007). Supported reflective learning: the essence of clinical supervision? Chp 2 in *Practising Clinical Supervision: A Reflective Approach for Healthcare Professionals* (2nd edition). London: Bailliere Tindall, pp. 27–50.

Gibbs, G. (1988). *Learning by Doing: A Guide to Teaching and Learning Methods.* Free on-line at shop.brookes.ac.uk

Kolb, D.A. & Fry, R. (1975). Toward an applied theory of experiential learning. In C. Cooper (Ed.), Theories of group process. London: John Wiley

Kolb, D.A. (1984). *Experiential Learning: Experience as the Source of Learning and Development.* Englewood Cliffs, NJ: Prentice Hall.

Lasswell, H. (1948). The structure and function of communication in society. In "The Communication of Ideas". Bryson, Lymon (ed). New York: Institute for Religious and Social Studies, p. 37–51.

MacLean, S. (March 2016, pp. 28–29) A new model for social work reflection: Whatever the weather. Professional Social Work. British Association of Social Workers

Rolfe, G., Freshwater, D., & Jasper, M. (2001). Critical reflection for nursing and the helping professions: A user's guide. Basingstoke, UK: Palgrave

Schön, D. A. (1983). The reflective practitioner: How professionals think in action. New York: Basic Books.

Schön, D. A (1991). *The Reflective Practitioner: How Professionals Think in Action Work-Base Learning a New Higher Education* (2003) Boud and Solomon.

Tuckman, Bruce W. (1965) "Developmental sequence in small groups." Psychological Bulletin, 63: 384–399.

7 Organisations and CPD

7.1 Introduction

Organisations within the UK construction sector can notoriously be difficult to define; on the one hand, a large construction company can be a principal or main contractor on one project, but on the other hand it can be the client owner on a speculative development site on another project. They can provide specialist services to a competitor and be required to procure and hire plant from their own in-house plant department. Further to this, larger companies will have dedicated Human resource (HR) departments, whilst the smaller companies may have a single person with some HR functions as part of the general administrative role.

This chapter looks at continuing professional development (CPD) activities of organisations within the built environment but in doing so attempts to unpick and clarify the aspect of the complex nature and relationships of those organisations. HR departments are identified as key to implementing recruitment and retention strategies and identify the workforce CPD needs, for example, through annual performance reviews or project-specific training needs. The industry professional bodies are discussed in relation to servicing the CPD needs of its members and others in the built environment.

7.2 The complex nature of construction organisations within the built environment

UK construction can often be viewed as a broad industry made of several different key areas, including buildings for housing, retail, and leisure; offices; hospitals; and schools. Larger civil engineering activities for utilities and infrastructure projects such as roads. Heating, ventilation, and air conditioning (HVAC) for buildings. Materials suppliers and manufacturers and a need for maintenance and repair sector across all projects. According to the Office for National Statistics' latest figures for 2018, the number of registered construction firms operating in Great Britain was around 325,736. The construction industry trade firms are given in Table 7.1.

This diversity across the industry allows competition to take place (Langford and Male, 2001), especially in sectors such as housing where entry requirement can be simply down to the availability of finance or the entrepreneurs' willing

Table 7.1 Construction industry trade firms

Main trade type: property developers	Main trade type: non-residential buildings	Main trade type: house building	Main trade type: civil engineering	Trade type: construction engineers	Trade type: demolition
Trade type: site preparation	Trade type: reinforced concrete specialists	Trade type: test drilling and boring	Trade type: roofing	Trade type: asphalt and tar sprayers	All trades: construction of highways
Trade type: construction of water projects	Trade type: railways and underground railways	Trade type: construction of bridges and tunnels	Trade type: construction of utility projects for fluids	Trade type: utility projects for electricity and telecoms	Trade type: construction of other civil engineering projects
Trade type: scaffolding	Trade type: installation of electrical wiring and fitting	Trade type: insulating activities	Trade type: plumbing and heat and air conditioning installation	Trade type: heating and ventilation engineers	Trade type: plastering
Trade type: joinery installation	Trade type: flooring contractors	Trade type: floor and wall tiling specialists	Trade type: floor and wall covering	Trade type: suspended ceiling specialists	Trade type: painting
Trade type: glazing	Trade type: plant hire (with operators)	Trade type: other construction work and building installation	Trade type: other specialised construction activities		

Source: ons.gov.uk Construction statistics annual tables.

to take a gamble in order to make a profit. Construction trades personnel are often employed on simple trade only contracts and materials tend to be fairly homogenous; for example, bricks of the same size across the UK, plumbing pipes, and fittings tend to fit in the same diameter sink holes and white goods tend to fit in the same standard 600 mm opening in kitchen base units. This allows for materials to be made cheaply through economies of scale distributed nationally and subject to competition.

The proportion of construction firms in the Great Britain in terms of the number of people employed can be seen in Table 7.2. At the smallest, Table 7.2 shows that 38,888 firms are sole proprietors and the largest 58 firms each employ over 1,200 staff.

The number of people employed either directly or indirectly in January–March 2020 by the construction industry was in excess of 2.3 million (ons.gov.uk/employmentandlabourmarket). This is a combination of craft, technical, professional, and managerial roles.

- The craft industry covers trade occupations including joiners, bricklayers, painters, scaffolders, roofers, and plant operators. Such trades are the constructors, assemblers, and finishers of a project.
- Technical occupations cover roles including architecture, site engineering, and site inspection. These provide the practical expertise to support the main professional such as the Architect and Quantity Surveyor.
- Professional and managerial positions include senior managers, site managers, Quantity Surveyors, and Architects. These roles are associated with the project team who design, plan, cost, and delegate work to project completion.

Table 7.2 Number of employees per type of construction firm

Size of firm (numbers employed)	*Number of firms*
0 (Sole proprietors)	38,888
1	138,069
2–3	88,297
4–7	35,434
8–13	12,890
14–24	6,444
25–34	1,939
35–59	1,932
60–79	556
80–114	474
115–299	554
300–599	145
600–1,199	56
1,200 and over	58
All firms	**325,736**

Source: ons.gov.uk construction statistics annual tables.

Broadly, the larger construction companies are mostly geographically scattered around major conurbations and often in overlapping market sectors. The type and size of construction projects aligns with the type and size of the organisation; the larger complex projects tend to be managed by large complex construction organisations and the mega projects through the creation of special purpose vehicles (SPVs). Specialisms such as ground works or heating often occur in niche areas to gain competitive advantage. Construction organisations will also employ technical and management professionals directly, through professional agencies, and on a consultancy basis. Table 7.3 identifies the types of professions employed:

The construction industry and the wider economy are often in a symbiotic relationship; for example, an increase in the demand for a certain good, say a new hybrid car, may provide a commercial opportunity for a car manufacturer to build a large new plant which will be built by a construction company. Competitors to the car manufacturers may then decide to follow suite so as not to lose customers and decide to modernise their existing car plants which will also use the services of construction professionals. These manufacturing decisions stimulate the construction industry and the construction activities of contractors all the way down the service and material supply chain, and the demand for raw material needed for building-related products is increased.

It is not limited to the manufacturing sector. The finance sector can do the same; for example, the Bank of England may decide to lower the base rate which in turn will influence the bank's interest rates. The lower the interest rates, the more willing a speculative builder is to borrow to build houses. Again, trades and material suppliers will be needed to service these new builds. Added to this, when

Table 7.3 Types of UK construction firm and technical and management professions

Construction project managers	*Architects*	*Site engineers*	*Site planners*	*Contract managers*	*Quantity Surveyors*
Architectural technologists	BIM managers	Building surveyors	Facilities managers	Town planners	Civil engineers
Process managers	Hydrographic managers	Geotechnical engineers	Service engineers	Health and safety managers	Logistics and supply chain managers
Package managers	Building inspectors	Highway engineers	Land surveyors	Asset managers	Structural engineers
Interior designers	Environmental specialists	Human resource managers	Cost consultants	Accountants	Marketing managers
IT managers	Financial managers	Hazard and risk managers	Project managers	Transport managers	GIS technicians
Buyers	CAD technicians	Estimators	Plant managers		

interest rates are lower, mortgage borrowing and house buying rise so the ripple effect can been seen in an increase construction activity.

Conversely, the repairs and maintenance sectors tend to increase when the economy is slowing down as borrowers are less likely to make large investments in new building and instead focus on repairing and maintenance of existing stock.

The construction industry is evidently a large sector of the economy and employs a broad and varied workforce of trade labour, technical staff, office administrators, and management professionals. The manufacturing and service supply chains directly or indirectly connected to the sector are also similarly made of a broad category of skills.

7.3 Workforce culture

The construction sector works within a dynamic framework for delivering projects to clients. This is typically formed from both a permanent organisation such as a main contractor and a separate temporary site-based organisation put together for a single purpose. This symbiotic relationship between permanent and temporary forms works because the industry is essentially project based; that is, it requires a permanent company to form a unique temporary group to come together in order to deliver a finished project, and after completion the group is disbanded, and the workforce and staff will move onto the next project. Obvious exceptions would be for design, build, finance, and operate (DBFO)-type organisation that employs its own staff and workforce. Even these will utilise the supply chain for special products and services.

Management and technical expertise tend to sit in a more centralised position with these types of organisational formations and will have control over trades and work packages. For that reason, deadlines and budgets are the normal metrics used to monitor and control construction work.

Balfour Beatty, for example, is a large public limited company (PLC) whose corporate headquarters are in London's Canary Wharf and employs around 26,000 people worldwide (balfourbeaty.com). It has regional offices, joint ventures, and associate interests throughout the UK and oversees across sectors of the construction industry. Such an organisation will undoubtably have its own organisational values and behaviours developed from its origins in 1909 by its founders George Balfour and Andrew Beatty.

Management thinkers such as Charles Handy and Edger Schien have studied organisational culture over many years and have well-known models of structures, behaviours, and values for permanent organisations such as Balfour Beaty. Values such as leadership, control systems, well-being, promotion opportunities, and training will be evident within its organisational culture model.

However, like most large and regional construction-related companies, organisational culture can be viewed from two aspects:

1 Permanent office-based staff
2 Site-based staff

Permanent office-based staff will typically be employed directly (or 'on the books') by the company and include office staff, accounts, administrators, HR managers, IT members, senior managers, and directors. The organisational culture of such an environment will have had time over a longer period to evolve, and its values and behaviours will determine the way its workforce is encouraged to develop. HR management (HRM) departments will have processes in place, and annual personal staff development reviews will be well established.

Site-based staff consist of management and the workforce. Management can be 'on the books' or project specific. Workforce can also be 'on the books' or be employed directly with a supply chain company. For staff and workforce not directly employed by the 'permanent' main contractor, its culture and values will be more fluid and more easily influenced by the smaller business owners, the team, or the type of trade. For example, on-site electricians may associate themselves with other electricians as they often share the same skill set and knowledge and often come across the same technical problems. Likewise, bricklayers may find that they share common day-to-day issues and therefore share common values. These common values from 'off-the-books'-type trades are shared across different projects as each moves around to find the work.

The size and turnover of single-person trades and sole proprietors are limited to hourly pay rates that allow for their own or family living expenses and perhaps a moderate disposable income. Consequently, annual staff development reviews do not form part of their formal internal business processes.

Consultancy-type sole proprietors differ; they can be a structural engineer, site surveyor, project manager, or cost and legal consultants, for example, employed on a project-by-project basis.

Organisations will often play a crucial role in developing an individual and organisational cultures often defined simply as "*the way we do things round here*" or more specifically defined in terms of shared values such as diversity and community and beliefs that provide norms that influence employee's behaviour. These norms often will include mechanisms for training and improving the skills of the workforce through mechanisms such as yearly reviews.

It could be argued that a temporary organisation such as those formed and based around a project will not have its own cultural history as it is a 'new' organisation. However, it will be made up of groups of individuals who have experience in these types of environments, and it is this regularity of behaviour which provides aspects of cultural norms (Ankrah et al., 2009).

Key factors that influence these types of organisational cultures include the following:

- The people – existing cultural traits
- Recruitment – selection based upon conducive behaviours and values
- Training – cultivating the desired cultural behaviours

The cultural dynamics of any construction project-based businesses will impact upon its ability to make a profit; therefore, employing the right people at the outset can be crucial. Consequently, retention in a short-term project-based organisation may not be subject to the same levels of scrutiny of those of a permanent organisation. Training budgets will also be subject to similar effects.

7.4 Human resource management

HRM has its roots in personnel management and covers the management of an organisation's personnel including those staff in the HR department. It also has a broader function of encouraging and maintaining shared values between the management and its workforce. Unlike personnel management, HR links the strategic aims of an organisation with the resources needed to help the management and workforce meet these objectives through training and development.

Consequently, HR departments will oversee the organisation's leadership, the organisational culture and ensure compliance with employment laws. The department is also responsible for:

- Attracting the right people
- Selection process
- Staff development and training
- Appraisal process
- Rewarding of employees
- Overseeing the well-being of the workforce

The transient and short-term nature of construction projects and workforce offers its own HR challenges, and it will include a continuous staff turnover and an ongoing skills shortage. The construction sector is often high risk with injuries and fatalities which necessitate comprehensive health and safety compliance procedures. The formulation of such health and safety procedures will stem from the HR department and be monitored by site management. Health and safety inductions and health and safety training will be mandatory for-site based personnel. Of all CPD training that is available CPD associated with health and safety is always considered the most critical.

A significant portion of the industry workforce is not employed on a permanent basis. This means many client organisations outsource for services such as specialist consultants and other niche service providers. Outsourcing to main or principal contractors is the norm, employed through tender and procurement contracts on a project-by-project basis; they themselves can also be considered permanent organisations with their own HR departments. Client HR departments work independently from the supply chain's HR departments.

7.5 Recruitment, development, and retainment

Strong positive cultures within organisations tend to attract career-focused talent. HRM covers the recruitment, development, and retainment of staff including the general workforce.

7.5.1 *Recruitment process*

The recruitment process attempts to create a pool of potential candidates from which a single applicant will be chosen. Once the job role description and specification has been written in compliance with current employment equality and diversity laws, it will be advertised internally within the company, externally outside of the company, or both depending on the type of job role, typically through the following:

- Recruitment agencies
- Professional journals
- The company website
- Universities' employability departments
- Online job portals

Applicants will normally be asked to complete an application form and/or submit a CV and covering letter and will be subject to an internal screening and selection process to reduce the numbers to a manageable pool of candidates. Some of the larger companies my use online tests or request the applicant to attend group and work simulation tests to reduce the numbers, some may conduct preliminary telephone interviews, and others may adopt all of these practices. Those candidates remaining will be asked to attend a formal personal interview and dependent on the nature of the job may also be required to deliver a presentation. HR will normally be present to oversee policy and employment law compliance and mitigate any unconscious bias or inadvertent discriminatory practices. HR can provide unconscious bias CPD training to remove unintentional stereotyping for those interviewing.

Once interviews have taken place, the interview panel will make their recommendation and the successful applicant will be given a conditional offer to the post subject to certain conditions such as adequate references or a medical for example.

7.5.2 *Successful interviews*

Successful applicants will normally:

1 Have a well-prepared and polished CV, and concise written covering letter
2 Be prepared beforehand by:
   a Understanding the job description and job specification
   b Researching the company
   c Dressing for the part
   d Being at the place of the interview at the correct time and before the start
   e Being prepared to answer and ask questions
3 Have made a good first impression

For the manager, the aim of recruitment is to attract the best possible candidates who will contribute to the organisation's strategic goals. Broader recruitment aims are to improve the business recruitment strategies, determine future requirements, and help attract the right candidates.

Recruitment agencies, mostly education establishments such as colleges and universities, will often provide CPD training for preparing for interviews.

7.5.3 Development and retention

Once the employee starts their role, the job of HR is one of retainment and helps in training and development. It is crucial for an organisation to hold onto its best and brightest employees as likely they may well be poached by competitors especially if the employee becomes disillusioned, feels undervalued, or is held back from any promotion and career goals.

Key retention strategies include:

- Appropriate reward mechanisms such as equitable salaries and bonuses
- Being valued in the workplace
- Healthy non-toxic office or workplace environments
- Training opportunities – in-house, on the job, or external programmes
- Career growth opportunities
- Promotional opportunities.
- A well-motivated workforce
- Leadership

Successful organisations will keep hold of their best employees through effective retention strategies; CPD training and development are a way in which to hold onto such employees.

Development is more than a short-term immediate skills update that shows immediate improvement in performance. Development concerns itself with future career growth. Development activities help in the broader problem-solving competences associated with management; for example, gaining a Quantity Surveying degree qualification brings specific technical knowledge associated with the role such as procurement and contracts. However, for the Quantity Surveying student engagement with the course over a three- or four-year period allows for learning and improvement of non-technical transferable skills such as:

- Working in groups
- Presentation skills
- Time management
- Written communication skills
- Problem-solving skills
- Learning other viewpoints

This type of long-term learning provides growth for the individual and benefits the company with a better highly skilled workforce able to work more effectively in groups, be creative in overcoming obstacles, better meet deadlines, and manage teams in often stressful situations.

Overall, the concerns of development and retainment stem from the recruitment function of an organisation. Many well-known and forward-looking construction organisations will already have strategies in place that allow for the integration between these three components, and it is for the career-focused individuals to recognise and seek out such companies. The need to oversee and manage staffing growth and performance often sits under the performance management function; this function helps HR and managers monitor and evaluate employees in order to meet the company's key strategic objectives as well as meeting the employees' own aspirational goals.

7.5.4 *Performance management*

Performance management is the function usually linked to HR that manages the employees in terms of their responsibilities to the organisation, motivation, skills update, and career goals. Managers will support HR in any implementation and monitoring strategies. Performance management will also imbue a sense of ownership for the employees who within this process take a lead in managing their own expectations.

Annual development reviews provide a useful starting point for performance management. However, short-term and intermediate goal setting, milestones, and tasked activities also form a crucial element to the function. For example, a manager may give ownership of a package of work such as procuring material on a project to a trainee, and the manager would guide and oversee the work progress to a satisfactorily end. The trainee will have gained some crucial experience of management work packages.

Performance management provides ongoing task and goal-setting opportunities for the employee with immediate feedback. For this feedback to be effective, it needs to be both consistent and effective, and this requires a certain type of manager. However, it would be wrong for a manager to expect an employee to perform on an activity that they do not have any meaningful knowledge or capacity to do and then receive negative feedback for failing to meet the required expectations; this will only disillusion the employee and may actually lead to them leaving. Managers would need the proper CPD management and mentoring training to support and encourage an employee, so it becomes evident that HR supports both the management and the workforce.

7.5.5 *Performance management system*

Performance management system (PMS) is a continuous set of processes developed to support the personnel towards the improvement of business performance and to the individual's growth. Some advocated benefits include the following:

- Holistic approach to improve performance and growth
- A useful diagnostic tool for identifying training and development needs across the business
- Identifying and rewarding talent
- A more engaged workforce

The system is developed, controlled, and monitored by HR with support at all levels of management.

Implementing a PMS will often take the form of the following four stages:

1. Plan – Agree and set measurable goals (using SMART methodology) with an employee.
2. Do – Make the goals part of any daily or weekly tasks.
3. Monitor – Monitor progress and give support, encouragement, and advice where necessary.
4. Review – Review if goals have been achieved, provide individual feedback, include any performance reward and then capture the lessons learned

This will involve the employee and manager sitting down and agreeing realistic goals at the outset. Any lessons learned after the activities have been completed would be used to support the individual in any new goal-setting strategies as well as general continuous business performance improvement outputs essential for business success.

Recognition of good performance can itself be a rewarding outcome to the employee and will often spur on further performance improvements. Rewards such as a financial bonus or a photo piece on the company's website or a team award will instil a sense of achievement and minimise dissatisfaction and at the same improve the employee's commitment to the company.

It is apparent then that performance management is a useful tool that supports the HR function in an organisation.

7.6 Annual development reviews

Annual development reviews, also known as performance appraisals or performance evaluations, form part of career development as well as a job performance review/reward mechanism. More recently, annual reviews have now become bi-annual six-monthly reviews, this reduces the likelihood of surprises and is a timely reminder of the agreements and objectives set at the start of the yearly review. Advocated benefits of annual reviews include but not limited to those in Table 7.4.

The review will normally consist of a single annual or six-monthly formal meeting that builds on earlier regular meetings and conversations that would have

Table 7.4 Benefits of annual reviews

Employee	*Organisation*
Identify achievements that contributed to the organisation's strategic aims	Improve the organisation's performance
Establish support for further individual development needs	Develop and encourage talent
Identify professional career development needs	Help meet the organisation's strategic objectives
	Retain high-performing individuals

occurred between the line manager and the employee. The key discussion points of the meeting will include the following:

- A review of previous objectives
- A review of performance and achievements
- An agreement of new or revised objectives
- A discussion on the means for achieving these objectives
- A discussion on personal career development aspirations

Performance review forms can be as simple as a single sheet of paper, with key sections that may include the following:

1. Employee information – name/role
2. Performance criteria – behaviours/strengths
3. Previous goals or objectives met/not met
4. Support – needs/requirements
5. New objectives agreed
6. Reviewer comments – signs off the agreed review form

For the employee, also known as the reviewee, the appraisal review forms are often partially completed by the reviewee prior to any meeting and then discussed with the reviewer and the review form fully completed and signed off within the meeting. It is important that the employee can talk about issues they feel pertinent to aspects of the review and respond to queries from the reviewer. In other words, it needs to be a fair open meeting.

A useful employee appraisal or performance and development review form may look like that in Figure 7.1.

The performance and development review form is used to measure and benchmark the employee's performance. The previous year's completed form will contribute to the appraisal meeting and help to evaluate achievements and any contributions made by the employee.

Rewarding performance gives recognition to those who have contributed to the company's goals and may include a financial bonus or lead to promotion with an increase in salary.

Performance and Development Review		
Reviewee: Employee Name		**Job Title**
Reviewer (Line Manager)		**Job Title**
Period under review		**Date of Review**
From:	**To:**	
Reviewee: Demonstrate any achievements (or training) within the period		
Reviewee: Summary of performance and achievements within the period		
Reviewer: Feedback - support given over the period – future expectation		
Reviewee: Future Goals (use SMART Methodology)		
Reviewee: Identify any training needs		
Reviewee Signature		**Reviewer Signature**

Figure 7.1 Employee appraisal review.

7.7 Personal development planning

Development planning allows the opportunity for the employee to discuss, plan and action career ambitions and opportunities. Personal development planning often forms part of any annual performance review and may be a separate document that will form part of the employees' personal career development portfolio. Personal development planning is discussed more comprehensively in Chapter 5.

7.8 Construction organisations and CPD opportunities

CPD events are often delivered at the place of work, either the head office or on site, also known as 'in-house' in medium to large organisations. At the behest of key senior management and technical staff, HR will often plan a CPD workshop around an identified need for some staff training and development. Typically, these can last from one hour to a few days and may be themed around the following:

- System and process updates, improving the way things are done
- Specialist software – upskilling and training
- Health and safety updates – first aid
- Legal updates – contracts and procurement

Staff can attend such events but need to be supported by their line manager, and these events are often linked to an employee's personal development strategies. In-house training can be more convenient as it means the employee is already familiar with the building and doesn't need to go to a new venue such as a training provider centre. In-house training also has the benefit of being more cost-effective as it saves having to send employees on training courses. Current professional staff can deliver these events, and where there is not a member of staff with the available knowledge, a third party can be contracted to supply the necessary training.

Professional bodies can play a very significant role in providing CPD events to members, and most are open to non-members as well. Table 7.5 shows examples of CPD events currently delivered by various professional bodies.

This table of CPD events provided by the industry professional bodies demonstrates only a small section of CPD activities available and delivered in the built environment, although the types of CPD activity will vary depending upon the type of learning and will normally take one of the following four simple forms:

1. Formal education and training – courses with assessments
2. Work-based or practice-based learning – on-the-job learning requirements
3. Professional events – conferences, workshops, and technical seminars
4. Informal self-directed learning – reading books and specific training manuals

There can be a further complexity of learning depending upon the sector of the industry, the organisation, and the nature of the CPD event.

There is a significant amount of CPD opportunities for anyone working in the built environment wishing to enhance their knowledge and expertise. For a

Table 7.5 Examples of CPD events currently delivered by various professional bodies

Professional body	*CPD event*	*Duration*	*Availability*
Royal Institution of Chartered Surveyors	Tendering Expert witness certificate Mediation training	4.5 hours 26 hours 50 hours	Members and non-members
Chartered Institute of Building	Alternative dispute resolution Leadership for high performance Becoming carbon neutral	2.15 hours 1 hour 1.5 hours	Members and non-members
Royal Institute of British Architects	Equality, diversity, and inclusion in business Designing for fire safety Managing client relationships	2.5 hours 2.5 hours 2.5 hours	Members and non-members
Chartered Institute of Procurement and Supply	Financial management for the supply chain Sustainable procurement Advanced negotiation	14 hours 7 hours 14 hours	Members and non-members
Association for Project Management	Introduction to earned value management Delivering engagement in integration webinar Women in project management conference	1 hour 1 hour 7 hours	Members and non-members

Table 7.6 Professional body's accredited courses

Professional body	*University degree courses*	*Duration (3–5 years)*
RICS	Quantity surveying Building surveying Real estate	Full time and part time
CIOB	Construction project management Construction management	Full time and part time
Royal Institute of British Architects	Architecture Architecture and environmental engineering	Full time and part time
Chartered Institute of Procurement and Supply	Logistics and supply chain management Procurement, logistics, and supply chain management	Full time and part time
Association for Project Management	Project management Programme and project management	Full time and part time

broader 'CPD' qualification, consideration should be given to a Higher Education vocational degree. Professional bodies accredit courses in their field for example (Table 7.6).

Table 7.7 Notional CPD outputs embedded with the modern apprenticeship

	Knowledge, skills (and behaviours) and CPD themes	*Evidence requirements and notional CPD outputs*
K1	Health and safety	Understand the principles and responsibilities imposed by law and other regulations in a construction environment.
K2	Sustainability	Understand the sustainability issues in projects across economic, social, and environmental aspects.
K3	Construction technology	Understand different construction techniques and materials and the principles of design.
K4	Contracts	Understand different forms of contracts used in construction and why they are applied in different situations.
K5	Procurement	Understand the different types of procurement process and negotiation requirements.
K6	Cost control	Understand the importance of controlling costs during a construction project and the effect of changes to the project.
K7	Financial reporting	Understand the various forms of reporting on project progress.
S1	Health and safety	Apply health and safety issues to all activities.
S2	Sustainability	Demonstrate application of the principles of sustainability.
S3	Construction technology	Assist in the implementation of the most appropriate solutions for construction projects.
S4	Contracts	Be able to apply different types of contracts to different situations.
S5	Procurement	Assist in the selection of and negotiation with specialist contractors for a construction project.
S6	Cost control	Assist in the measurement and costing of construction works during a project.
S7	Financial reporting	Assist in the preparation of financial reports, cash flow, and cost forecasts for a construction project.
S8	Administration	Assist in the collection, collation, and storage of relevant data and its analysis.
B1	Commitment to code of ethics	Understand and apply the Code of Conduct and conduct regulations, ethics, and professional standards relevant to industry's recognised professional bodies.
B2	Continuing professional development	Identify own development needs and take action to meet those needs. Use own knowledge and expertise to help others when requested.
B3	Commitment to equality and diversity	Understand the importance of equality and diversity and demonstrate these attributes so as to meet the requirements of fairness at work.
B4	Communicate effectively	Be able to contribute effectively to meetings and present information in a variety of ways including oral and written.
B5	Conflict avoidance	Be able to assist in planning to avoid conflict and resolving issues that do arise.
B6	Work in teams	Be able to work with others in a collaborative and non-confrontational way.
B7	Demonstrate innovation	Be able to identify areas for improvement and suggest innovative solutions.

As well as higher degree qualifications to support personal development the UK government's new modern apprenticeship schemes combine work with study. For those embarking on a modern apprenticeship programmes, it can be seen that inherent within the course outcomes model are built-in knowledge, skills (and behaviours) (KSB)-type outputs which can also be considered as a structured approach to achieving an intermediate range of CPD goals culminating into a degree qualification.

For example, those who want to become a Quantity Surveyor may prefer the modern apprenticeship route and need to be successful in applying for the post with a construction organisation to apply to go on a course. Once employed the organisation may already have a partner or if its new to them will partner with a Higher Education supplier, i.e. a university, which will facilitate the required learning and end qualification.

In this instance for a degree in Construction Quantity Surveying demonstrates the required notional CPD outputs embedded with the modern apprenticeship framework (Table 7.7).

The framework shows 22 knowledge, skills, and behaviour elements and demonstrable CPD themes that need to be delivered and evidenced on completion of the course. One clear advantage of this route is the link to professional body registration as the final assessment process will, as advocated by the Institute for Apprenticeships and Technical Education, "typically be partly representative of the review process required for professional registration".

7.9 Conclusion

This chapter has identified the diverse nature of organisations within the UK construction industry. The range of companies and the sectors have been ascertained and shown that the number of firms and those employed directly or indirectly contribute significantly to the UK economy.

Construction organisations have a propensity to have their staff operating on two fronts: permanent head office staff and a transient site-based work force. Consequently, working relationships and separate cultural norms become evident in the way people work together and in their long-term goals.

HRM covers all the permanent and temporary employees of the organisation and ensures compliance with employment law, recruitment, and retention as well as the well-being through personal development as evidenced through annual staff reviews.

These reviews form the backbone to the employee's CPD goals for those who wish to achieve growth and promotion opportunities. Professional bodies provide a plethora of CPD and training courses for both members and non-members. A further and broader development for employees is through the degree or modern apprenticeship routes. These qualifications can be seen inherent within them to offer a range of themed CPD activities over a longer period and are linked to professional chartered membership.

References

Ankrah, N., Proverbs, D. and Debrah, Y. (2009). Factors influencing the culture of a construction project organization: An empirical investigation. *Engineering, Construction and Architectural Management*, 16(1), 26–47.

Langford, D. and Male, S. (2001). *Strategic Management in Construction*. 2nd ed. Oxford: Blackwell Science.

8 Managing the CPD of others

8.1 Introduction

An important aspect to managing the continuing professional development (CPD) and personal development of others is to keep them motivated. Human resource management and management principles should therefore include encouraging the workforce to develop in their role. There are demonstrable benefits to the individual and the organisation which have been dealt with in Chapter 7.

Organisations' mentoring strategies can provide such encouragement and focus and organisations' wishing to invest time in the workforce. The role of mentoring is explored in this chapter, and reference is also given to the role of professional bodies in mentoring candidates.

8.2 The role of mentoring

The role of the mentor is to guide a less experienced individual, for example, in their own career development. A good relationship is considered essential, and mentors who also see themselves as reflective practitioners often see this as a mutually beneficial endeavour. It is a long-standing and well-developed tool for supporting personal development.

There is often confusion between coaching and mentoring; both concepts attempt to help in the development and improve the learning of the individual. However, both have clear differences in the way they are used and when they should be used. Table 8.1 shows the way these differences fall into common themes:

The choice the individual makes of when to use a coach or mentor depends upon the individual or the organisation's needs; both can overlap and will support the individual in a number of different ways.

A coach is more appropriate if:

- You need to develop a new skill in a short period of time.
- You need to improve your competencies.
- You need new knowledge to suite a new situation.

Table 8.1 Key differences between coaching and mentoring

Theme	*Coaching*	*Mentoring*
Purpose	Improve personal or work-required efficiencies, enhance current knowledge, or achieve new skills	Continuous improvement of the individual A more holistic approach to career development
Timing	Short term. Can be as little as a few hours or a few days	Medium to long term. Can be a few years or lifelong
Structuring	Clear and regular, structured, scheduled meetings with an end date or on the accomplishment of a specified outcome	May start formal, develops into more ad hoc schedule of meetings as needed by either party
Leadership (expertise)	The expert 'Coach' is normally hired for a fee and attempts to develop or update specific skills of the participant	Mentors are typically in a position of seniority in a specific professional area in the organisation or to the individual. Helps to influence and develop the individual to meet their own goals
Goals/outcomes	Outcomes are clear, pre-defined and measurable. The coach may be involved in developing the outcomes and the coaching method need to meet the outcomes	May be more fluid as the relationship develops over time. Path to achieve goals may change and develop Development of the individual's competencies and reflective skills is of more interest.

Attending specific CPD events can satisfy these requirements such as attending an asbestos awareness training course if your company is planning to work in the refurbishment sector. Where such programmes are not available bespoke programmes can be created with the aid of specialist consultants. For example, your organisation may be implementing an in-house quality system and staff need specific training.

A mentor is more appropriate for:

- Membership of a professional body such as the Chartered Institute of Building (CIOB) and the Royal Institution of Chartered Surveyors (RICS).
- Internal career development
- Leadership development
- Succession planning

Your organisation may require an individual to have full membership of a professional body to gain career advancement for example from Assistant Quantity Surveyor to Quantity Surveyor, or for succession planning an organisation may decide to encourage junior management into senior management roles and a

Table 8.2 Approaches and traits of mentoring

Approaches	*Traits*
Classic mentoring	Wise and trusted sage-like
Leaders	Inspire to succeed
Models	Role models provide examples to emulate
Coaches	Educate and equip
Teachers	Share knowledge, inspire to learn
Advisers	Advise on specialist knowledge
Counsellors	Listen and non-directive
Buddies	Buddy system, assigned to help newcomers

Adapted from Pegg (1999).

senior director may wish to mentor a certain member of staff for future a leadership role. Other reasons to use mentoring include the following:

- Supporting existing staff with new roles
- Supporting new starters to an organisation
- Supporting CPD

According to Pegg (1999) in *The Art of Mentoring*, good organisations will define what a mentor should and should not do, i.e. clarity is vital. Approaches to mentoring are provided in Table 8.2.

Good mentors have different strengths and different approaches to mentoring but in the main will have a combination of the above traits. For the organisation, the benefits of mentoring include improvement in:

- Skilled workforce
- Recruitment and retention
- Job satisfaction
- Productivity

According to Clutterbuck (2004), to the individual the benefits can be seen as:

1 Increased confidence and self-awareness which helps build performance
2 Development outcomes
3 Better management of career goals
4 Developing wider network of influence

There are many suggested ways to mentor an individual. Alred et al. (1998) suggest a simple three-stage model for mentoring. The model can be used as a plan of action in a mentoring meeting. Although it is possible to use the model over a number of meetings rather than doing the three stages over one meeting, it can be used to identify single action issues that can be progressed and actioned. Here

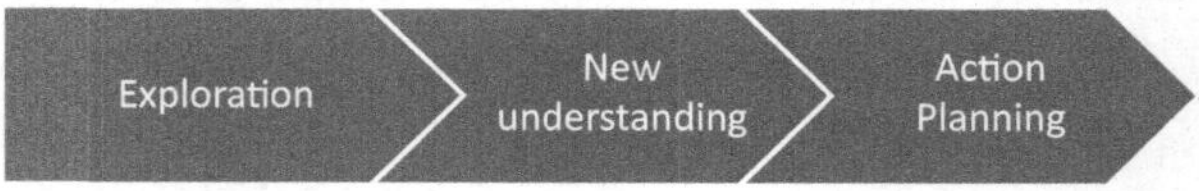

Figure 8.1 Exploration, understanding, and planning.

an issue could be simply giving help in finding a way to support or identify some personal development training for the individual being mentored (Figure 8.1).

Application

1 **Exploration** – Explore the issues identified by the mentee. The mentor helps and encourages the mentee to open up and talk about the issues important to the mentee.

The mentor's role – Take the lead in any discussions and encourage the mentee to come to their own answers. Listen, support, and pay attention. It is important not to rush as important aspects may be overlooked.

The mentee's role – Try and be clear and articulate on issues. Be honest and be prepared to discuss things that are important to your growth and development. Talking to a mentor can help identify the trivia from the significant.

2 **New understanding** – Once the relevant issues have been identified, the mentee is encouraged to reflect and consider the wider context of the issues as this may provide a new perspective. The mentee is also encouraged to consider what is delaying any growth and development opportunities.

The mentor's role – Support and understand. Make constructive comments and give constructive feedback. Recognise strengths and identify development needs. It is useful to share experiences but do not make the focus on you. Identify and agree the development needs.

The mentee's role – You should begin to discover new perspectives on issues, and you may begin to rethink your role which can be uncomfortable. New learning may take place and you should begin to recognise the potential for going forward in new and revitalised ways.

3 **Action planning** – Set specific actions to work on in achieving new goals. Focus on solutions and build upon positives.

The mentor's role – Be prepared to listen and encourage the mentee to think about options. Steer the conversation towards action planning specifics such as goals, time, and how the mentee will overcome any barriers.

Help set a realistic action plan and agree an achievement date followed by a progress meeting or a next meeting date to discuss the achievement.

The mentee's role – To be creative and brainstorm for solutions. To establish achievable goals and action plans that suite your own circumstances.

Mentoring is not often clear-cut, and it can mean going back to the start a few times part way through the process. The primary relationship in mentoring is between the mentor and the mentee. However, if the process goes back to stage 1 to many times, you need to question the validity of the mentor/mentee relationship.

8.2.1 *The GROW model*

Developed originally for coaching the GROW model by John Whitmore in his book *Coaching for Performance* (1992) is a method for setting goals and problem-solving, and can be used in mentoring conversations – specifically as a structured approach in more formal meetings and conversations between the mentor and mentee. The model can be viewed in cyclical form (Figure 8.2).

Application

1. Goal – Help the mentee to set sessions goals at the start of the meeting and establish their long-term aspirational goals.
2. Reality – In order to help the individual it is crucial to identify the experiences, knowledge, and skills they have and the experiences, knowledge, and skills they need to achieve their long-term goals. Discussion around staff appraisal results and/or other feedback from HR and line managers can help to establish the mentee's current position. This requires the mentee to be honest and realistic.
3. Obstacle/options – Based upon establishing the mentee's current position, short-term goals can begin to be established. Discussions around the

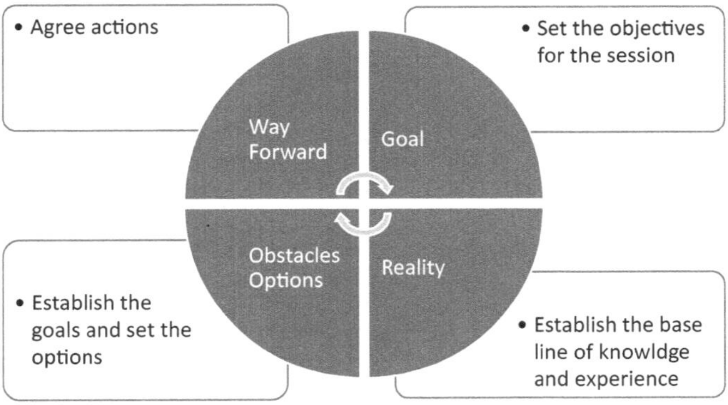

Figure 8.2 Grow Model adapted from Whitmore (1992).

likelihood of achievement of each option and how they will know that they have met these goals should be considered. These questions should be answered.

4 Way forward – A plan of action is established including support needs and progress reporting. Application of SMART goals is useful here.

Both the mentor and the mentee should be aware that the process is not set in stone and there is the possibility that some discussion points and content can often overlap. Many practitioners will list the questions to be asked in each stage of the GROW model which can often be useful. Table 8.3 includes examples of the type of questions that will help the conversation in the meeting.

The GROW model is well established across several industries and one of the most widely used models. It is considered successful in attaining leadership and management goals. A GROW model mentor/mentee meeting form example is given in Table 8.4.

This form can be used when the meeting is taking place in a more formal pre-agreed session; this allows ideas and brainstorming to take place free from work distractions.

There are other models such as TGROW, CLEAR, OSCAR, OSKAR, STEPPA, and ACHIEVE.

Table 8.3 Typical mentoring GROW model questions

	Key themes	*Sample questions that can be asked*
Goal	What do you want?	1 At the end of the session, what do you like to have achieved? 2 What would you like to discuss? 3 Why do you want to achieve this goal? 4 Are you able to take ownership of yourgoals?
Reality	Where is your current situation?	1 Is this an accurate assessment of your position? 2 Do others agree with what others think of this assessment? 3 What steps have you already taken? 4 What do you think I can do for you?
Obstacles – options	What can be done?	1 What is preventing you? 2 What would you do if the obstacle is not in your way? 3 How can you reach the goal? 4 What could be your first step?
Way forward	What are your next steps?	1 Can you commit to a realistic plan of action? 2 When will you know you have reached the goal? 3 When shall we have our next meeting? 4 When will you start your plan of action?

Table 8.4 GROW model mentor/mentee meeting form

Mentor mentee meeting form		
Mentors name:		Mentees name:
Session no.		Session date
Goal		Comments
What is your:	Session goal? Short-term goal? Or Long-term goal?	
Reality	What is a realistic assessment of yourself?	
Obstacle	Why can't you achieve your goals?	
Options (can be more than 1)	How can you reach your goal(s)?	Option 1 Option 2 Option 3
Way forward (Select the most realistic option)	SMART goal setting	

Table 8.5 TGROW model

	Key themes	*Sample questions that can be asked*
Topic	Broader themes should be discussed.	1 What would you like to discuss? 2 Why is this important to you? 3 What do you want to gain from this?
Grow	Setting specific goals	See the above GROW model for details.
Reality	What is the mentee's current situation, and what needs doing?	
Options	Exploring different options to achieve the goal	
Way forward	'Agreeing action'	

8.2.2 The TGROW model

The TGROW model builds upon Whitmore's GROW model. This model follows the same sequence except another stage that is added to the start. Developed by Myles Downey (2014) in his book *Effective Coaching: Lessons from the Coaches' Coach*, Downey believed that the Topic at the outset is needed so broader issues are discussed that would help set the context when setting specific goals (Table 8.5).

The model is more fluid than the GROW model because there are fewer specific questions that need to be answered at each of the CLEAR stages. This model can be used either when management believe improvement will help the individual or when an individual is looking for development growth.

Table 8.6 CLEAR model

Contract	For the mentor and mentee to reach an understanding and develop an agreement. Key discussion points include setting the boundaries or scope; establishing the desired goals for both parties; and agreeing the timing, length, and venue of meetings.
Listen	Active listening can often be a difficult process. It can be about picking out feelings, themes, and messages from the mentees and requires active listening. The mentor should be encouraging conversation and be attentive and empathetic. Questions of clarification can be asked to encourage openness.
Explore	The mentor begins probing with the aim to get the mentee to make a realisation of the problem or the obstacle. The mentor can challenge feelings and assumptions to raise more self-awareness.
Action	The start of the journey to reaching the goal. Commitment from the mentee is required. A structured plan may be developed by the mentee supported by the mentor. Options are narrowed down to single route to the goal.
Review	A review of the session is done to remind of both commitments, support strategies, and understandings. Short follow-up meetings are arranged to support the progress being made by the mentee. Positive feedback through this is essential so as not to demoralise the mentee if progress is slow.

This model helps when there are a lot of influences and dynamics going on in the life of either the mentor or the mentee. At the second stage of discussions, agreements are as Whitmore's GROW model.

8.2. *The CLEAR model*

The CLEAR model was developed and expanded upon by Professor Peter Hawkins in publications such as Hawkins, P. and Smith, N. (2013). *Coaching, Mentoring and Organizational Consultancy: Supervision and Development*. The model framework is given in Table 8.6.

8.2.4 *The OSCAR model*

The OSCAR model was developed by Andrew Gilbert and Karen Whittleworth and can be found in their book *The OSCAR Coaching Model* (2009). This model builds upon the GROW model and can be a useful choice for mentors. It creates a framework for questions to be asked in the mentor/mentee meeting although the questions are not necessarily structured so moving backwards and forwards in the stages is possible. The model builds on five connected stages and is presented in Table 8.7.

The model is useful for mentors who prefer a more participatory relationship with the mentee. The mentee will take ownership of their own development and growth whilst the mentor will provide support.

Table 8.7 OSCAR model

	Key themes	*Sample questions that can be asked*
Outcome	Focus on the aims and goals of the session. Clarify outcomes.	1 What would you like to achieve from this meeting? 2 What is your long-term goal? 3 What do you want to achieve and how will you know that you have achieved it?
Situation	Evaluate the mentee's current situation to enable the mentee to go to the next stage.	1 What is your current situation? 2 What are the issues impacting on your situation? 3 What are others saying about your current situation?
Choices	Determine options to explore and consider the consequences of choosing each option.	1 What are your options that will help resolve the issue? 2 What are the consequences of doing these options? 3 Which of your options has the least impact on others?
Actions	Consider the steps needed and preferred option and develop a detailed plan of action.	1 What actions will you undertake? 2 What support will you need to help you? 3 On a scale of 1–10 how motivated are you to do this action?
Review	Develop a clear review process and agree a regular or milestone meeting schedule.	1 How will you review your progress? 2 Can we agree a meeting schedule? 3 Are the actions moving towards the results you want?

8.2.5 The OSKAR model

The OSKAR model was developed by Mark McKergow and Paul Z. Jackson and expanded upon in the publication *The Solutions Focus: Making Coaching and Change SIMPLE* (2007). The model is essentially a coaching framework but can be applied in both coaching and mentoring situations, and it can also be used within a team or within the organisation to help improve specific performance issues. The model is an alternative to others and is advocated to provide a focus on helping in positively changing the mentee's behaviours which require help in improving their own development and growth (Table 8.8).

The model is a collaborative approach to mentoring and allows the mentee to determine success. The focus of the model is on its approach in using small steps and as such quick gains can be achieved. Having a clear personal outcome or goal helps keep a focus for the mentor and mentee. The model provides a useful set of tools for a busy mentor.

8.2.6 The STEPPPA model

The STEPPPA model was developed by Angus McLeod and expanded upon in his book, *Performance Coaching Toolkit* (2010). This model is used to provide a

Table 8.8 OSKAR model

	Key themes	*Sample questions that can be asked*
Outcome	Understand the purpose of the session and what the mentee wants from the session.	1 What do you want from this process? 2 What is your goal? 3 How will you know this session has been a success?
Scaling	Establish how close the mentee is to achieving the goal.	1 Can you rate yourself today on a scale of 0–10 to where you are in relation to achieving the goal (where zero is as far away as is possible)? 2 Can you provide evidence to support your scaling position? 3 How long would it take to realistically get where you want to be?
Know-how	Identify the needs gap and identify key support or resource requirements.	1 What existing strengths do you have that will help? 2 How do you know these existing strengths will help? 3 What support do you need to make an improvement?
Affirm and action	Positive feedback to affirm what has been achieved and focus on the next step.	1 In terms of making small steps, what has gone well so far? 2 What actions did you employ to see this improvement? 3 What is the next step?
Review	Continuous review of progress and improvement position.	1 What progress have you made? 2 Do you need to further support or resources? 3 How are you applying this growth?

useful means for mentoring and specifically as a prompting tool during the mentoring session and as a reflective tool post-session. It is a useful framework for dealing with the emotional element of a problem or barrier. Details of the model are given in Table 8.9.

Emotions can be both the biggest motivator and the biggest demotivator; this model attempts to reinforce the motivational commitment made by the mentee throughout the mentoring programme. The overall aim of this model is to keep the mentee engaged with the process using an emotional investment framework.

8.2.7 The ACHIEVE model

This mentoring and coaching model was developed by Fiona Eldridge and Sabine Dembkowski from their observations on coaching practices in 'Beyond GROW: A New Coaching Model', *International Journal of Mentoring and Coaching*, vol. 1, issue 1, Nov. 2003. The authors argue that the model is a logical extension to Whitmore's GROW model. The ACHIEVE model is normally presented as a cyclical process and focuses on seven key stages where the last stage feeds back into the first. Table 8.10 provides a useful application of the model from the mentor's perspective.

Table 8.9 STEPPPA model

	Key themes	*Sample questions that can be asked*
Subject	Establish the agreed topic under consideration in the mentoring programme.	1 What would you like to discuss? 2 What do you want to focus on? 3 Will your focus have an impact on the organisation?
Target identification	Refine the discussion towards an achievable goal.	1 What outcome would you like to be by the end of this session? 2 What are your short-term and/or long-term goals? 3 Do you have a timeline for achieving your goal?
Emotion	Establish the key emotional driver which will underpin achieving the goal.	1 On a scale of 1–10 where 1 is not very much, how much do you want your goal? 2 What would make you more motivated? 3 What would achieving this goal look and feel like?
Perception and choice	Establish conscious perception. Develop an understanding of the context of mentee and its wider impact. Consider routes to success and make choices.	1 What do perceive to be your current situation? 2 What is the current barrier to achieving your goal? 3 Is this the correct target?
Plan	Develop a clear plan of action.	1 Is the plan achievable? 2 Does the plan feel right? 3 Does the plan conflict with aspects of your organisation?
Pace	Structure paced-out plan with periodical and timely review of progress.	1 What would be a realistic time frame? 2 Can you put progress reviews in place? 3 Will you need support?
Act/amend/adapt	Establish a workable plan of action. Get commitment from all stakeholders.	1 Are you ready to go ahead with the plan? 2 What did you get out of the session? 3 Are there any barriers remaining and how will you overcome them?

This model has its roots in the workplace and as such provides a realistic mentoring model. It is possible to repeat the process if at the final stage an alternative strategy is required to enable the mentee to achieve their goals. Other models include the following:

- The CIGAR model – Suzy Green and Anthony Grant (2003)
- The LASER model – Graham Lee (2003)
- The ARROW model – Matt Sommers (2004)

Table 8.10 ACHIEVE model

	Key themes	*Mentors action points*
Assess the current situation	Develop an understanding of the mentee's current state.	1 Be able to ask the right questions. 2 Listening skills. 3 Establish a rapport and a genuine sense of connection.
Creative brainstorming	Stimulate open discussions. Widen the mentee's current perspectives.	1 Challenge the mentee's current position. 2 Explore different possibilities to growth and accomplishment. 3 Develop a sense of possibilities.
Hone goals	Convert possibilities into a set of goals.	1 Be explicit in what is not wanted as well as what is wanted. 2 Consider the application of SMART goal- setting methodology.
Initiate option generation	Generate options for goal achievement.	1 Assist in aiding the mentee towards generating several general options. 2 Makes sure these are the mentee's choices.
Evaluate options	Scrutinise and prioritise options.	1 Encourage the mentee to develop their own set of ranking criteria for evaluating the options. 2 Keep a decision matrix for each option.
Valid action plan design	Design a valid action plan, and add depth and structure to the preferred option.	1 Get the mentee to commit to their plan. 2 Consider and agree what the first step is. 3 Agree the support needed to achieve the goal.
Encourage momentum	Provide ongoing support and agree progress meetings	1 Encourage and motivate the mentee. 2 Give positive feedback.

- The PRACTICE model – Stephen Palmer (2007)
- The POSITIVE model – Vincenzo Libri (2004)
- The OUTCOMES model – Mackintosh (2005)
- The STRIDE model – Will Thomas (2005)
- The GENIUS Coaching model – Alec McPhedran (2006)

Mentoring and coaching are well-developed forms of training and development for supporting personal development. Any chosen model should be tailored to the type of mentor and the type of mentee. Consequently, the number of mentoring models available is vast and can be overwhelming to the new mentor. Not only should the mentor and mentee match, but both should be matched with an appropriate model that provides the best help to achieve their goals. For the mentor, these goals may well be to simply provide support for someone else's growth and development.

8.3 Professional body's mentoring requirements

The construction industry's professional bodies will have as part of their internal support frameworks mechanisms for mentoring for membership, personal development, and CPD. These 'mentors' are not always defined in terms of mentors but still provide the same or similar supporting roles.

8.3.1 Royal Institution of Chartered Surveyors

RICS guidance and assistance strategies take the form of an Assessor. The assessor's role applies to:

1. Reviewing candidate's submission documentation
2. Preparing competency-based questions
3. Participating in assessment panel interviews
4. Contributing to the decision-making process
5. Contributing to candidate feedback

However, the RICS Assessment of Professional Competence (APC) pathway can provide candidates with a supervisor and a counsellor. This type of mentoring can give the candidate up-to-date insights, advise, and give guidance on the APC content. It can also offer encouragement and support on presenting and writing leading up to the final assessment interview.

To become a mentor, applicants are encouraged to attend the APC Supervisor and Counsellor training course. The advocated learning outcomes according to the APC Supervisor and Counsellor Guide are that the mentor will be able to:

- Describe the different stages of the APC process.
- Identify the role, responsibilities, and requirements of the supervisor, the counsellor, and the assessor.
- Differentiate between AP competency levels: 1 – knowledge and understanding, 2 – application of knowledge, and 3 – depth and synthesis of technical knowledge and implementation.
- Illustrate what the RICS expects the trainee to be able to demonstrate at the Final Assessment and what they need to do to prepare.
- Explain what the assessors are looking for during the Final Assessment.
- Demonstrate the assessors' questioning style.

Third-party coaching services for Assessment of Professional Competencies will also provide mentoring services. These third-party service providers will often include qualified RICS assessors.

There is no formally agreed mentoring structure advocated by RICS. Instead mentors are left to provide their own guidance.

8.3.2 Chartered Institute of Building

For non-members or those at the final stage to gaining full chartered membership, a Professional Review (PR) is often the final action prior to full membership. Candidates often require support and the institute provides local workshops and mentoring services to give guidance on your PR application.

This mentoring framework is known as a PR Support Provider, which is a network cited by the institute as 'trusted individuals and organisation' providing support and encouragement through the application process.

The CIOB provides guidance on the process through a PR Support Provider to mentor a candidate, which is taken from https://www.ciob.org/professional-review:

1 The candidate needs to contact a PR Support Provider (from a detailed list of training addresses provided) and appoint someone you feel happy to work with.
2 Once appointed, your PR Support Provider will give you encouragement and support via workshops or other method of digital media.
3 After your initial session, you will be asked to submit your application to your provider. Your provider may suggest some revisions giving you the opportunity to strengthen your application. You will be given timescales and encouragement to help you stay on track.
4 The provider will make an assessment of your PR application and submit on your behalf to CIOB.

Within the institute the mentoring process is clearly limited to the full membership application process and the mentoring role is not particular detailed. Once becoming a full member, there are no further formal structured mentoring schemes available.

8.3.3 Association for Project Management

For routes to full membership, there is no evidence of any structured approach to formal mentoring or coaching opportunities for the candidates.

Work-based learning mentoring may have taken place for those candidates working in the field of project management, or for those with a formal qualification, academic mentors may have provided support to the individuals whilst studying for their award.

8.3.4 Institution of Civil Engineers

The Institution of Civil Engineers (ICE) mentoring platform is an online service that helps members with their professional development by matching each with suitable mentees and mentors. Table 8.11 identifies the advocate benefits to both parties as detailed by ice.onpld.com.

Both parties need to register online and choose a path as either a mentor or a mentee. Once registered, the mentee can use the online service to find a mentor from a list. Those mentors with the specific skills and experience that the mentee

Table 8.11 ICE mentoring platform

Advocates' benefits for having a mentor	*Advocates' benefits for mentoring*
Receive independent advice about your expectations and professional development.	The ability to develop your coaching and mentoring skills, which can contribute towards your CPD plan
Develop the capabilities and skills needed to succeed in a dynamic global economy.	The ability to pass on your experience as an employer or employee
Identify your strengths, weaknesses, and the best way to use these in your civil engineering career.	A chance to use your communication and leadership skills and industry knowledge
Studies show that professionals who have a mentor earn more annually than those who do not, and 75% of interviewed executives say mentoring has played a key role in their careers.	The satisfaction of helping others enhances their career development strategies
Gain insight into the different routes available to achieve your career goals.	A new perspective on your professional and personal experiences
Develop knowledge of discipline-related and non-technical skills, which could contribute towards your CPD plan.	Satisfaction from helping others to overcome challenges and in this way broadening your own experience
Access support, professional development, guidance, and networking opportunities.	The opportunity to develop new skills through the process of 'reverse mentoring'.

values are identified, and the mentee then sends a request to be mentored. Once accepted, the mentoring activities will start, goals will be created, and progress reviews will occur to review milestones and achievements. It is wise to select and apply one of the coaching/mentoring models discussed earlier. Once the process has been fully completed and the goals have been met or if the process is terminated, the relationship will formally end.

ICE mentors also provide guidance on mentor-supported training for trainees wishing to become members and who require a different type of guidance through their Initial Professional Development (IPD). This IPD sets the required attributes needed for applicants prior to becoming full members. To become a mentor in mentor-supported training, an online application is required to be completed including ICE membership details, evidence of qualifications, CPD records, and a CV. These types of mentors are typically middle or senior managers.

8.3.5 *Chartered Institute of Procurement and Supply*

Chartered Institute of Procurement and Supply (CIPS) mentoring schemes in respect of the four routes to full chartered membership:

1 Studying for CIPS professional qualifications

This is a CIPS exam-based route – no evidence of any formal mentoring or coaching opportunities for the candidate embarking on this route to membership.

2 An accredited degree

This is through accredited university degrees and programmes – no evidence of any formal mentoring or coaching opportunities for the candidate embarking on this route to membership.

3 The CIPS Management Entry Route (MER) for senior professionals

Designed for those with extensive experience in the field and who operate at a senior strategic role and assessed through an online questionnaire – no evidence of any formal mentoring or coaching opportunities for the candidate embarking on this route to membership.

4 The CIPS Corporate Award

CIP offers a range of applied learning programmes, with assessment-based outputs to that help individual meet all the programme's aims and objectives – CIPS programme management team works with the individual and provides mentoring support.

There is little evidence of mentoring support in the route to full membership except for those embarking on the CIPS Corporate Award.

8.3.6 Royal Institute of British Architects

The Royal Institute of British Architects (RIBA) Professional Experience and Development Record (PEDR) as stated by RIBA is "a digital record of a student's experience, development and competency in the practice of architecture".

For those wishing to become an architect in the UK, registration through RIBA is mandatory to complete Part 3 requirements of 24 months of practical experience recorded online on RIBA's own PEDR platform. Students must register onto the systems to access the platform. This is followed by the Part 3 exam.

Mentoring takes place supporting the student over this 24-month period and is specifically applicable to the employment mentor. RIBA sets out the criteria to be a supervisor:

- The individual who directly supervises the student
- Has detailed professional knowledge of the work prepared by the student undertaking professional experience.
- Should be an architect with at least five years' experience of the design of buildings and the administration of subsequent contracts.
- An experienced professional in their own field and, if possible, a member of an appropriate professional organisation.
- May not necessarily directly employ the student.

The mentor's advocated role is to:

- Directly supervise and have detailed professional knowledge of the work prepared by the student undertaking professional experience.
- Support the student during the practical experience to gain the professional knowledge and skills typically required for working in the architecture industry.

- Review and approve the students' logged or record sheet online, following completion of a short appraisal with them to offer feedback and plan for the next quarter.
- Provide constructive and evaluative feedback for the student.

RIBA considers the students who are under direct supervision by the employment mentor and defines direct supervision as "*a person/professional supervising the student who should have responsibility for and control over the work being undertaken. Direct supervision does not mean the employment mentor has to necessarily employ the student*". Essentially, RIBA provides a clear definition and a structured role for the mentor. The requirement goals for the candidates are also defined, and mentoring is mandatory.

8.4 Conclusion

Mentoring has been shown to be a useful tool for developing a person's skills and knowledge beneficial for both the organisation and the individual. Mentoring models allow mentoring to take place in a structured way. There are several existing mentoring models used across many sectors, most notably health care and sport. This seems to be where most mentoring models have been developed, sport will use 'coaching' models that are transferable to be 'mentoring models'. For the 'new' mentor there is a wide selection of choices, and for the mentee knowing these choices is useful as they will be able to select a model most suitable for them. Of the construction professional bodies that offer aspects of mentoring, perhaps the most useful one was the ICE-advocated mentoring model. The institution comprehensively demonstrated its commitment to its members

References

Alred, G. & Garvey, B. (1998) Mentoring and the tolerance of complexity, in: European Mentoring Centre, 5th Conference Proceedings, Burham, UK.

Alred, G., Garvey, B. and Smith, R. (1998). *Mentoring Pocketbook*. Alresford: Management Pocketbooks.

Brockbank, A. and McGill, I. (2012). *Facilitating Reflective Learning: Coaching, Mentoring and Supervision*. 2nd ed. London: Kogan Page.

Clutterbuck, D. (2004). *Everyone Needs a Mentor: Fostering Talent in Your Organisation*. 4th ed. London: Chartered Institute of Personnel and Development.

Clutterbuck D., & Megginson, D. (2004). Techniques for coaching and mentoring. London: Butterworth-Heinemann

Dembkowski, S. & Eldridge, F. (2003). Beyond GROW: A new coaching model. The International Journal of Mentoring and Coaching, 1(1), November.

Downey, M. Effective Modern Coaching: The Principles and Art of Successful Business Coaching; LID Publishing Ltd.: London, UK, 2014; pp. 73–84.

Gilbert, A. &Whittleworth, P. 2009. The OSCAR coaching model. Simplifying workplace coaching. Monmouthshire: Worth Consulting Ltd.

Hawkins, P and Smith, N. (2013) Coaching, Mentoring and Organizational Consultancy: Supervision and Development

Jackson, P.Z. & McKergow, M. (2007). The Solutions Focus: Making coaching and change simple (2nd ed.). London/Boston: Nicholas Brealey

McLeod, A., & Thomas, W. (2010). Performance coaching toolkit. Maidenhead: Open University Press.

Pegg, M. (1999). *The Art of Mentoring.* Industrial and Commercial Training, Vol. 31(4), MCB University Press, 136–141.

Whitmore, J. (1992). Coaching for performance: A practical guide to growing your own skills (People Skills for Professionals). London: Nicholas Brealey Publishing.

9 CPD examples from other industries

9.1 Introduction

This chapter explores the professional development practices of organisations from both the construction industry and other industries, such as banking and finance, software and manufacturing. Some of the practices undertaken by companies from different industries are discussed. These are used as fictionalised examples of the practices that are currently undertaken to provide inspiration for companies and professionals looking to develop their own CPD practices. Many companies have several CPD initiatives but only a brief selection are utilised in this chapter to illustrate the different, and sometimes similar, approaches companies from different industries may take to CPD. The inclusion of these approaches to professional development, taken from wider industries, is in the hope that industries can learn from one another for the greater good of all staff – and that the construction industry in particular can learn from the best initiatives other companies, both in and outside of the construction industry, can offer. In this chapter there are many different techniques and programmes discussed; some of which overlap with those already employed by the companies operating within the construction industry. Other initiatives mentioned are currently not widely used, and so could be directly transferred and used by construction companies in their current format, or certain elements utilised and developed further to make the initiatives more applicable to the construction industry whilst ensuring the core advantages remain the same. The overriding theme in this chapter is that professional development does not have to be a solo journey, and you can be helped on your way by the organisation you work for. If your organisation does not offer any support, development, or training, then it may be worth considering your future at that organisation, or at least discussing with the appropriate management some of the practices described below. The company may be more than willing to help you develop by providing innovative and exciting opportunities. This could lead to your current company adopting aspects of those tried and tested development initiatives discussed, as the company will then ultimately receive the benefits of having a highly developed workforce. With all that being said, the conclusion of this chapter does reiterate that the ownership of personal and professional development is firmly at the feet of the employee. You cannot and should not rely solely upon your company to take responsibility for your own development. If your company does take development seriously then that is beneficial to both you and them. If they do not, and won't adopt any of the practices discussed, then CPD will have to be gained elsewhere.

9.2 The construction industry

9.2.1 A *leading Multi-Disciplinary Consultancy* (A)

A leading international publicly listed Multi-Disciplinary Consultancy company that offers design, planning, and consulting services across construction, engineering, and infrastructure. This consultancy is the result of many mergers although can trace its heritage back over a hundred years. Merges ultimately result in different company approaches and values coming together and, in this case, have successfully resulted in a numerous development initiatives offered to staff.

One training and development initiative offered is a Graduate Development Programme which aims to develop both the soft and technical skills of recently graduated staff. It is a two-year programme including induction days, residential training events, support towards professional accreditation, mentoring, on-the-job training to improve technical development, external training courses, and support and advice on continuous professional development (CPD) throughout a graduate's career. There are also guidance books produced for all employees that provide a wealth of professional development information and encourage proactive practices such as setting goals, identifying career pathways, and arranging ongoing discussions with line management. There is also a company 'University' and an adoption of the 70/20/10 split approach to development, with 70% of an employee's development coming from on-the-job training, 20% through coaching and mentoring, and the final 10% from formal learning.

9.2.2 A *leading Multi-Disciplinary Consultancy* (B)

A design, engineering, and project management consultancy that focusses on the energy, infrastructure, and transportation sectors. Again, a company with over 100 years history but has been the subject of mergers and acquisitions over its lifetime. This company serves customers worldwide.

A flagship Graduate Development Programme is aimed at recent university graduates and is a training framework that lasts three years. During this period employees develop their skills and knowledge across several disciplines with a focus on becoming chartered with a relevant professional body. The programme consists of mentoring, on-the-job experience, and specific training modules. You will also regularly meet up with other graduates on designated events and learn about other parts of the business via internal work placements.

9.2.3 An *international main contractor* (A)

A large construction company with a long heritage that operates internationally. This contractor offers a range of services across the whole project lifecycle on a wide range of infrastructure projects. With over 20,000 employees worldwide focussing on core business segments the company puts great emphasis on staff development.

Understanding that their reputation and ability as a company is built upon the abilities of their staff the contractor empowers all employees to take control of their own career direction and support a 70/20/10 professional development split. This is where all professional development undertaken is broadly 70% on the job, 20% learning from colleagues, and 10% of your time is spent on training courses and more formalised learning events. The contractor understands that development is ongoing throughout the entire careers of their employees, and so have development programmes in place for staff that come with regular development progress reviews. Support is also offered to allow employees to become chartered with the relevant professional body. The company has in place a set of highly important modules available to all staff and also more specialised programmes covering topics such as inclusive leadership and emotional intelligence for those employees wanting to develop into future leaders.

9.2.4 *A national consultancy*

A UK-based national consultancy that specialises in the residential development and the investment market. The consultancy frequently contributes to and publishes industry-leading publications on how the construction industry can and should improve to be ready for future challenges. They are focussed on enabling employees to have the skills, attributes, and competencies to professionally develop as the consultancy understands that by inspiring their employees, employees will in turn inspire clients.

The consultancy has a clear set of values for all staff and focusses on providing support to all employees to develop their skills and knowledge in cost and project management, supply chain and purchasing, development expertise, and contract administration. The consultancy also aims to build a value-driven collaborative and supportive culture and engage in a diverse range of team building initiatives. This includes holding regular quiz nights, supporting staff volunteering activities and an exercise and yoga programme to help relieve stress and increase mindfulness. The initiatives undertaken are often summarised in a regularly published online newsletter. It is through the development of a creative, collaborative, and supportive office atmosphere that the consultancy allows its people to professionally develop.

9.2.5 *An international main contractor (B)*

An international main contractor, engineering and asset management company with a heritage that can be traced back nearly 200 years.

This main contractor heavily invests in the development of their own staff with a focus on building the skills and leadership qualities required to meet the future needs of the construction industry. The company has a focus on schemes that combine on the job development through experience with more formal academic qualifications. They also have learning and development support networks that identify and fast track future leaders into managerial positions within the business.

9.2.6 A *national main contractor*

A national main contractor with numerous business units that again has a heritage spanning nearly 200 years old and a billion-pound turnover. Personal growth is linked to employee's well-being and the contractor has received numerous awards for staff development. Over one-third of employees have taken part in some form of development, with the company having an online brochure of training courses for all employees to select and complete, including on topics such as health and safety, managerial training, technical knowledge, and sustainability. The company also supports all employees in having regular performance reviews and aims to deliver training to employees that is above the industry average.

The main contractor also has a 12-month leadership programme aimed at maximising the management potential of employees. The programme is also academically accredited allowing employees who complete it to have credits towards achieving a Masters qualification. They also have a Management Trainee Programme that pairs trainees with mentors allowing bespoke development plans to be in place to identify and support specific training needs, as well as allowing Management Trainees to work across all areas of the business to increase their future leadership knowledge and ability.

9.3 The banking and finance industry

9.3.1 A *large international bank (A)*

One of the UK's largest banks with headquarters in London, but with worldwide operations across a range of financial services.

This bank has several skills development programmes in operation, aimed at a wide range of individuals including graduates, ex armed forces, and apprentices. The bank places a large emphasis on its staff development, with a bank-wide learning and development programme. This programme focusses on making CPD flexible and fit the time and development needs of staff. The programme is governed by a framework of values including under which sit initiatives and concepts that ultimately aim to embed key leadership values across the business. The framework also sets out percentages that can be broadly correlated to the amount of time total development will come from different sources. For example, 10% is formal. It is envisaged staff will get 10% of their development from formal sources such as technical training, education providers, professional qualifications, or based on leadership curriculum. 20% is social. Development will be achieved from mentors, peer-to-peer learning, and speaker sessions from senior leaders. Finally, 70% is experiential. This is where development will be achieved from desktop training, interactive online content, regular feedback, and immersive skills and leadership experience. This is the same 70/20/10 approach that is adopted by many companies across different industries.

9.3.2 *A large investment bank*

An investment bank and financial services provider that employs over 40,000 people. The bank offers extensive online learning and business podcasts that are available to all staff even new recruits before they officially commence employment. At each employee's different career milestones, programmes focussing on leadership and culture are tailored to meet their individual needs. Nearly every employee also completes at least one hour of classroom based or digital training each year.

Feedback 360 is another initiative the bank offers. This allows any employee at any stage the opportunity to either request from, or give feedback to, colleagues. It is aimed at enhancing relationships, improving performance, and understanding where to focus development. There are also training programmes aimed at specific employees within their organisation including bespoke and innovative leadership development programmes. The bank also has an in-house University which aims to provide development opportunities at every stage of an employee's career. This includes offering training and programmes on a wide range of areas and topics to suit the immediate and future needs and ambition of all staff members.

9.3.3 *A large international bank (B)*

Through a combination of growth and acquisitions this bank is one of the largest banking institutes in the UK and a largely recognised and respected banking institution internationally. The bank has regular planned meetings between staff and managers where clear career development goals are set. Working together, managers will help members of staff identify and plan how to help staff become more effective in their professional role, offering detailed feedback along the way. Each member of staff is also encouraged to take personal responsibility for ensuring they meet personal development targets. Additionally, the bank also has internal mentoring and buddy schemes, the latter of which provides an experienced member of staff to act as a buddy to answer any questions from the new graduate scheme intake.

The bank also has an in-house University where staff members are able to access online courses that they can complete at their own pace, with courses aimed at communication, leadership, and presentation development. Courses can be linked to the member of staff's current role, a role they aspire to achieve, or courses the bank thinks are important based on the members of staff location and level.

9.4 The food and drink services industry

9.4.1 A *fast-food company*

This company also has an in-house University that started life as a training programme that was ultimately focussed on educating and developing employees on the correct methods of running a successful restaurant. The development programme now offered consists of a comprehensive positive-focussed approach to the development of all staff. The company prides itself on promoting from within and having a high investment spend on staff development.

One programme offered is linked to a part-time degree, includes block week study, and allows employees to experience every aspect of the business, so employees can build on the business theory they gain and apply it to the business itself.

9.4.2 A *leading UK supermarket*

A leading supermarket that has diversified over its lifetime, so much so that to put it under the food service heading is doing the company a great disservice in failing to acknowledge the wider market interests such as banking, insurance, fuel, clothing, and energy just to name a few.

As the winner of numerous awards for staff support and development the supermarket has development strategies that offer staff externally accredited training and apprenticeship programmes. They have a leadership programme that encourages staff to pursue charitable endeavours, and also have their own training college aimed at team leaders and store managers to help enhance technical and behavioural skills.

9.4.3 A *leading drinks manufacturer*

With over 200 drink brands available across more than 180 countries the organisation has been involved in mergers, acquisitions, and business unit sales to grow to its current size with a focus on core business models.

The manufacture seeks to empower their staff to enable them to become the best they can. They do this with a focus on areas of importance including the development of skills and entrepreneurship through their own Academy. This Academy offers online learning resources with a focus on the functional development of employees. The company also undertakes annual reviews that aim to provide detailed feedback and forward-looking career guidance to staff.

9.5 The software industry

9.5.1 An *international software company* (A)

A company that arguably operates in every country and has pioneered many software advancements since its inception that dictate and guide the way modern-day businesses operate. The company has many staff development programmes that all put employees at the centre of its approach as they believe solid business foundations are achieved when employee development needs are met. The approaches adopted by the business value learning over knowing with their training philosophy to provide the correct learning via the best method at the appropriate time. The company also offer customised manager training with the aim of enhancing mentoring and coaching skills, frequent promotion opportunities, and classroom learning opportunities.

The company invests in many development programmes including an apprenticeship programme aimed at recruiting developing and training non-traditional talent. This programme combines hands-on project experience with classroom learning and allows the applicant to select a tailored and focussed apprenticeship pathway based on their own experiences and ambition.

9.5.2 *An international software company* (B)

An international software company with more than 20,000 employees that is regularly voted one of the best companies to work for. Guided by its core values to everything it approaches the company has achieved pay parity across all employees in location and job role regardless of gender or ethnicity. Whilst this may not appear to directly link to the professional development of staff it is of the upmost importance. If every employee does not feel like they can progress professionally at the company they currently work, they will look to leave. This is even more compounded if employees feel their lack of progression is due to factors based on ethnicity or gender, for example, as no matter how hard they develop their skillsets and experience, they know they will not be able to progress. So aside from all the negative legal, ethical, and reputational factors involved in not ensuring parity amongst staff, ultimately an organisation that does ensure parity, or have a real plan in place to achieve it, is less likely to retain staff.

For specific professional development the company empowers staff to manage their own development, with the assistance of several employee development programmes such as a learning fund. This allows employees to be reimbursed up to an annual set threshold to take advantage of educational and learning opportunities and offering all employees a set amount of funding to be used on personal growth and development opportunities such as conference attendance and short courses.

9.6 The manufacturing industry

9.6.1 A *leading car manufacturer* (A)

At the start of 2020 the manufacturer directly employed over 40,000 staff members across the world. The company has a blueprint that represents what they stand for, as well as their passions and values, and these are communicated to all stakeholders.

As part of their professional development skills programme, set up to help managers deliver inspirational leadership and improve professional growth, the company focusses on a few main areas. These include identifying skills gaps, analysing how these skills gaps can be addressed, delivering the required training, and ensuring all interventions are aligned with business strategies.

Personalised development plans are also requested from staff that allow employees to discreetly select from a modular plan to enhance their own skillsets in a shorter, specific, and more focussed method. The programme now has over 50 courses aimed across the managerial disciplines and includes development areas such as emotional intelligence, commercial acumen, and financial management. These are all engaging and innovative and designed to replicate real-life situations managers may face. Such courses also include the use of actors, role-play scenarios, and self-study toolkits. To date the programme has impressive completion and feedback amongst staff and has been recognised in leading industry awards.

9.6.2 A *leading car manufacturer (B)*

One staff development initiative of this leading manufacturer is aimed at students. This is an intensive training and development programme that seeks to equip students with the required skills for a successful manufacturing. The programme adopts a blended approach to staff development, of classroom-based theory (delivered through partnerships with colleges), hand-on laboratory exercises, and self-paced learning. The manufacturer has also adapted the programme into a shorter taster course that can supplement younger student studies to bridge the gap between formal education and full-time employment.

9.7 The power and infrastructure industry

9.7.1 A *leading services and communications company*

One of the world's leading communications services companies founded over 150 years ago and operating in nearly 200 countries. This company has several values which guide their practices, as well as a successful and renowned graduate scheme. The company also encourages graduate communities run by staff that contain a wealth of information and promotes wider discussions and networking.

The graduate programme focusses on the actual role the employee is being hired to fulfil. The programme is very orientated towards a real work-based learning environment with every employee on the graduate programme undertaking a 'real' role in business. This is buttressed with wider training and development opportunities throughout the duration of the programme that are aimed at personal and professional improvement across many criteria. This includes critical and commercial thinking, team working, problem-solving, and customer relationships.

The company also has an Academy that is open to all employees across the business at every level and is focussed on aiding staff in their professional development. This includes the creation of a career map that helps identify all the required skills of future roles so employees can map themselves against them in order to understand where they need to develop in order to progress.

9.7.2 *A major infrastructure, transportation, and power company*

Over 150 years old this company has changed the world in which we live across many industries and sectors, and invests heavily in employee development.

This investment includes a focussed curriculum that trains over 150,000 global supply chain employees for the future. The course is also available for all employees to undertake if they desired and is a tailored receptive programme that meets individual needs through hands-on training, immersive boot camps, and a range of online courses. The focus of the programme includes advanced manufacturing, digital technologies, and lean manufacturing. The programme itself consists of an online course, advanced workshops, academy-based training, and an immersive leadership programme.

9.7.3 *A leading energy services company*

This company focusses on coal, oil, gas, onshore, deepwater, and low-carbon energy solutions. A global energy company based in London, this company operates at nearly all levels of the industry from exploration of raw material to production, distribution, and marketing. The company has a wealth of programmes and initiatives to assist employee development including a mentoring facility, structured online courses, graduate programme, and future leaders programme which focusses on identifying enthusiastic leaders and giving them the required skills and opportunities to lead the business in the future.

The company also aim to build the enduring capability of all employees and so launched an in-house University to provide a development framework for all staff. This is online and consists of different group-wide academies that focus on different business unit requirements. The aim of the University is to make learning flexible and fun. This company also takes the approach that 70% of an employee's development will occur through on-the-job experience, 20% via relationships, and 10% through formal educational training. The development initiatives also focus on building presentation and communication skills, technical abilities, and leadership and management development, and are available to all staff at all stages of their career.

9.8 The retail and clothing industries

9.8.1 *A leading sport brand*

The aims of the company include a focus on enhancing the working environment, building a performance culture, and being a company of choice. The company believes that all employees need a training plan and a mentor to help develop strengths and overcome challenges. A performance culture amongst all employees is encouraged that consists of leadership, performance, and talent management. Elements of these programmes include measuring and evaluating an employee's current performance against the job role they are undertaking. As an employee's performance is ultimately linked to their remuneration results an employee's performance management evaluation will be used to determine their financial compensation. The evaluation tool also includes learning, training, and development requirements aimed at performance improvement across both an individual and a team level on concepts such as the managing of people, team development, and strategic management.

9.8.2 A *leading adventure brand*

One initiative of this adventure brand is to connect staff with brand ambassadors on teambuilding trips away. These can include hiking, skiing, and climbing across terrains throughout the world. Teambuilding exercises such as these bring all staff together and encourage bonding, and help build relationships and trust in ways that are difficult, if not impossible, to simply build on the shop floor, or office environment, alone. More formal development initiatives offered include instructor-led and online learning programmes, staff coaching, career planning and goal setting, and performance managemént exercises.

9.8.3 A *national services outlet*

With over 5,000 UK staff this national company has a wide business focus and provides all employees with the resources they require to develop their career. They expect all employees to utilise these resources and maximise the opportunities provided. These include the provision of a mentor to all new employees, and then a week-by-week training plan that supports employees to develop. This plan is also linked to financial rewards in that every skill an employee gains increases their bonus potential. There are also in-depth practical training guides provided for all staff with a focus on 'on-the-job' training and development.

9.9 A summary of development initiatives

The following training and development initiates have all been discussed in this chapter alongside the type of company that embraces them. However, they are repeated in Table 9.1 for ease of consideration, and to provide an informal checklist for what companies can and do offer for the professional development of employees.

Table 9.1 Training and development initiatives

• 360 Feedback	• Immersive training opportunities	• Reflection processes to identify gaps in current knowledge
• Apprenticeship programme	• Induction days	• Regular feedback meetings
• Blended learning	• Initiatives to improve company culture towards supportive development	• Residential training events
• Buddy schemes	• Internal training courses	• Self-titled 'University' or 'Academy' that houses all company training materials
• Company training brochure	• Internal work placements.	• Seminars
• External training courses	• Leadership programmes	• Shadowing colleagues and peer-to-peer learning
• Flexible learning	• Learning fund available to employees	• Skill development programmes
• Formal external academically accredited courses	• Measurement and evaluation of current performance	• Staff coaching
• Formal externally delivered training courses	• Mentoring	• Support towards professional accreditation
• Goal setting workshops	• On-the-job training	• Teambuilding activities
• Graduate Development Programme	• Online material and courses	• Training plans

9.10 Analysis of professional development initiatives

All the company types discussed in this chapter offer some sort of training and development to their staff. For some, it is a more formal and long-term development strategy, whilst for others the development has a more short-term and immediate focus. From analysis of each company's learning, teaching, and development initiatives several 'insights' can be gained. These can help companies be authentic in their development practices and provide a checklist for employees as to what to look for when working at, or considering working at, different employers at different career stages.

9.10.1 Insight 1: Values

Analysis reveals that the majority of companies have some form of a mission statement, with values and often published company aims that drive the company culture. These are utilised to ensure consistency and focus, and so all stakeholders are aware of what the company stands for. Whilst some companies may have such things and not enact them in an authentic way, these companies will often be 'found out' and their true motivations revealed, resulting in adverse publicity and a de-motivated workforce with a high number of staff turnover. However, having company values and staying true to them will help guide an organisation in the right way, to make the right decisions. Where these values directly reference and impact upon the company employees, and the company employees believe the values are authentic, a collaborative and supportive organisational culture is fostered.

It is always worth checking as an employee or potential future employee, what a company's values are, and if you can find evidence of these in the company itself through articles, reports, or word of mouth. If a company has values in place, that are actively and actually lived on a day-to-day basis, this could lead to a more positive and focussed development culture and could be a good place to work to develop your own skill sets and knowledge in the short-term and potentially offer a rewarding and challenging career long-term. As a company, if your competitors have values in place, that are authentically enacted and promoted, and you do not, you may find it difficult to compete in securing motivated employees who want to professionally develop, and so ultimately suffer commercially.

9.10.2 Insight 2: Development for all

The development opportunities on offer are usually available to all employees, although some initiatives may be focussed on some employees over others, such as a graduate scheme. Companies will generally have training and development opportunities of some degree for all their staff (or at least should have). This can be an ad-hoc approach to development as and when it is needed (when a new contract is won, or when a new member of staff joins to company) or it can be a more formalised and structured approach to development, with every employee having to complete certain development requirements on an annual basis. This also largely depends on the organisations size, and some larger companies have self-titled programmes to deliver development, whereas smaller companies do not have the resources to create such marketing worthy development programmes. However, as graduate schemes appear to be so prevalent in the industry amongst larger companies, it is worthwhile for companies of all sizes that operate in the construction industry to be aware of such programmes. If a similar initiative can be introduced it could be beneficial from a recruitment perspective with attracting future professionals. Programmes such as 70/20/10 are also widely used which promote a varied approach to staff development utilising both internal and external resources.

If a company is going to provide some support with employee professional development, somewhat regardless of scale, they need to offer comparable development opportunities to all staff in order to continue the culture of development and training for all, and in order to ensure all staff are fully trained and ready to provide the best services they can to customers and be as effective as possible. From an individual's perspective, no matter how well the company has helped develop your skills and knowledge previously, if such opportunity or support stops when you reach a certain position, often what is the motivation keeping you at the company? It is always wise, however, to realise that at some hierarchal levels (i.e. graduate) you may receive more direct guidance and development from a company then when you reach certain other levels (i.e. manager). However, you should still receive the opportunity and support to develop further, even if not in such an overt and formal manner.

9.10.3 Insight 3: Availability of opportunities

The initiatives companies offer should also be available on a flexible basis. Each employee will have a different preferred method of learning and training. Whilst it is not possible to make every initiative available via multiple delivery methods, several initiatives delivered via different methods should be an organisational aim. For example, some employees may prefer structured face-to-face classroom-based formal training, whereas other employees may prefer the exact opposite, with flexible online-based informal opportunities. If an organisation can offer multiple training methods for employees at each level, including face to face; online; team orientated; working alone; internal, external and blended initiatives, then no employee will be left behind.

9.10.4 Insight 4: A two-way relationship

It should also be noted that all companies that have a focus on the professional development of their employees will expect this development to be a two-way relationship. No company will invest time and resources into the development of employees, if those employees do not take advantage of the opportunities offered, and do not show motivation and commitment to development. If this occurs a company may be less likely to invest in the development of staff. This relationship also works the other way, in that if an employee is highly motivated and committed to professional development, but an employer offers no support, the employee may consider that it is not the best environment for them to work in and look for employment elsewhere.

It is therefore a balance that is required, between the support offered by a company and the motivation and willingness of an employee. It is important this balance is realised, understood, and addressed so that both parties are aware of each other's requirements and expectations. This could be formalised in a learning agreement or embedded in the organisation's culture and values. Either way, it is of paramount importance for both an employer and employee to be aware of the reciprocal relationship required for both to prosper.

9.10.5 *Insight 5: Professional accreditations*

Many learning, training, and development initiatives offered by companies are accredited by third parties. This could be an internal training course externally accredited or external short-, medium- and long-term courses such as apprenticeships and degree courses.

Professionally accredited external formal courses need to be balanced with internal and informal courses, to suit all employees' preferences and requirements. However, there is a trend amongst companies to help support employees, particularly graduates, towards a professional accreditation. This is beneficial for all employees, as a successfully completed externally accredited course of any duration, is something that employees can take with them if they were to transfer employment. That is not to say companies should be used by employees for training and development purposes only, and then leave to seek employment elsewhere; in some respects, construction is a small industry and how professionals portray themselves is of the upmost importance. But employees do change employment for a variety of reasons and having professionally accredited qualifications is arguably more likely to open more doors of opportunity in the future.

9.10.6 *Insight 6: Mentoring*

Mentoring is probably one of the most commonly utilised initiates when it comes to employee development. It has many advantages over other methods. First, companies are full of experienced and helpful employees who will want to work with other, most likely newer, employees. The frequency by which meetings can occur and the personal and applicable experience that can be conveyed, as well as the increased networking and team building associated, are all hugely beneficial. This form of development is also very cost-effective as it involves no externally paid training providers and can be built into the job specification of existing managerial level employees.

9.10.7 *Insight 7: Feedback*

Feedback can take many forms but always plays a crucial role in professional development. Whether from the perspective of employees or an employer, a manager or someone being managed, giving and receiving feedback is ultimately key to improving skillsets and knowledge. We need to know things have gone right, and why they have, and if things could be improved and how. If you simplify many development initiatives, they are all just different methods of feedback. An action is carried out, the inputs and the results are reflected upon, feedback is then received and hopefully analysed with relevant actions undertaken. Feedback in relation to professional development is explored in greater detail in Chapter 8. However, is it worth reiterating, companies that are successful in the professional development of employees, and individuals who are effective at developing professionally, all understand the importance of feedback.

9.11 Conclusion

This chapter has summarised different development initiatives that can be used by companies across all industries. Companies often have more than one initiative aimed at the CPD of its employees, and often these overlap between companies, with one company offering a similar CPD initiative to another. There are also bespoke approaches to CPD adopted by some companies, with innovative and effective initiatives designed and delivered to ensure employees are continuously developed. Nevertheless, some companies may not offer such a range of CPD activities. It is clear to see, however, that no matter the industry, professional development of employees is taken seriously by most, if not all, type of companies.

The summary of development initiatives will hopefully serve as important examples about what companies can offer so that other companies can learn and adopt similar practices. These are presented in an effort to illustrate the range of development practices currently occurring in other industries. By doing so, it is hoped construction companies of all sizes can find inspiration for the creation of a new staff development programme, or simply gain reinforcement for the programmes they have in place. Individual construction professionals should also be aware of what other companies offer for professional development of their own staff, in case their current organisation does not take professional development of its staff seriously.

Finally, it is worth stating that all development is a two-way relationship. This is evidenced more overtly in some initiatives than it is in others, but the expectations still exist. Construction professionals require organisations to take employee development seriously and provide suitable support and opportunities. Organisations in return expect employees to take advantage of the opportunities provided and commit to taking part in development initiatives with motivation and enthusiasm. If this two-way relationship breaks down it can be unfortunate for all parties, employees will not want to work for a company that does not support them to develop their skills and knowledge, and companies will not want members of their workforce to not take advantage of the professional development the company offers.

It is also worth noting that where companies fail to provide adequate support and opportunity for staff to develop, it is the responsibility of individual professionals to ensure their own skill sets and knowledge are suitable for both the responsibilities they currently have, and the roles they aspire to hold.

10 Why construction professionals need to take responsibility for their own career development

10.1 Introduction

The chapters of this book have shown that the construction industry significantly contributes to the UK economy. However, when compared to other UK industries, the construction industry has been described as having a 'productivity problem'. The following is a brief summary of some of the research included in this book and how the role of CPD can help professionals develop their own skills and careers and by doing this also go some way to addressing the larger issues experience in the built environment today. An industry report by the professional body the Chartered Institute of Building (CIOB) described the construction's 50-year battle against low productivity and stated that when compared to other industries, and even against other countries' construction industries, employees in the UK appear to work longer hours simply to produce an equivalent economic output (CIOB, 2016). Most studies and industry reports that have attempted to investigate this 'productivity problem' have taken a macro-level analytical approach, where any analysis has tended to focus across the broader economy and all market sectors. There is, therefore, a gap in current research on productivity in construction from a micro-level analysis perspective. Micro-level analysis is concerned with small parts of the economy and can be viewed as a local-level, small group, or even individual phenomenon. It is argued that a micro-level analysis needs to consider a unit of measurement lower than an individual organisation, such as its staff, with the approach being described as necessary to understand productivity growth (Carlsson, 1987).

Carlsson (1987) also states that economic competence should be assessed at both an individual level and an organisational level and argues the productivity of individuals is directly linked to the wider productivity of the organisation. In turn, it could be argued that the productivity of individual organisations within a single sector ultimately contributes to the overall productivity of that industry. In the construction industry, however, there exists a gap in understanding concerning a micro-level analysis of the built environment professionals' level of productivity and how this is impacted by their organisation's behaviours. As part of this book research was undertaken that sought to address this gap and consider the links between the perceived self-productivity of construction professionals and the continuing professional development (CPD) practices of their employers. If an organisation understands how it can improve the productivity of its staff, then it will inevitably be able to increase its own productivity and in the process perhaps improve the productivity of the wider construction industry. By exploring this gap in current literature, this research also sought to identify areas for future research and provide recommendations regarding the directions this future research could pursue.

10.2 The construction industry and its productivity problem

The UK construction industry contributes over £99 billion per year, some 6.5%, of the UK economic output (ONS, 2017; Rhodes, 2019). It is argued that the industry improves the very fabric of society (Glass and Simmonds, 2007) and includes the design, construction, management, and demolition of buildings, infrastructure, and engineering projects. As of Q2 2019 there are over 343,00 companies and 2.4 million employed by the construction industry in the UK representing 6.6% of people in employment (Rhodes, 2019). The contribution, therefore, of the construction industry to the UK economy can be classed as significant.

Despite this significance, the construction industry has, however, always experienced what has been called a 'shortermism', where the individual and organisations that make up the industry only focus on short-term profitability at the expense of long-term investment and value. It is argued that this has contributed to the industry's 'productivity problem'. The Office for National Statistics (ONS) is recognised as the UK's largest independent producer of statistics and reports directly to the UK Parliament. The main responsibility of the ONS is to collect, analyse, and disseminate statistics regarding the UK's economy, society, and population. The ONS produces all relevant and applicable productivity information, which is measured as output per hour and is expressed in pounds per hour of output. Data from the ONS reveals that the average productivity of the whole economy has only marginally improved between the periods of Q1 2007 and Q4 2017 from £32.5 to £33.7. In the same time period, the construction industry has improved from £24.0 to £27.0. However, this is still far below the average of the UK economy. Such figures look especially worrying when you consider the services sector, manufacturing, production and agriculture, and the finance sector, which all outperformed the construction industry across the same time period.

To address the 'productivity problem' of the construction industry, the UK government released an industrial strategy in 2013 entitled 'Construction 2025'. The strategy also aimed "to put Britain at the forefront of global construction" and outlines five broad aims. The Construction 2025 report, as well as its five aims, is explored in greater detail in Chapter 2. The first of these aims is to be an industry known for its talented and diverse workforce. In order to achieve this, a greater investment is needed in the development of that workforce. This was echoed a few years later in 'The Farmer Review of the UK Construction Labour Model: Modernise or Die Tie to Decide the Industry's Future' by Mark Farmer. This report highlights how low productivity is a symptom of the construction industry and calls for stronger leadership, training, and investment in development to tackle this issue (Farmer, 2016).

However, as the industry is made up from so many disparate companies, which often are competing against one another, it can often be difficult to encourage enough collaboration to arrive at a consensus so that a single unified voice can represent the industry by speaking on its behalf. Nevertheless, there have been attempts to unify the industry's voice with differing levels of success. Whilst many professional bodies exist to represent sectors of the industries or individual professions operating within it, there have also been attempts to create forums representing the professional bodies themselves. One example is that of the Construction Leadership Council (CLC) (explored in greater detail in Chapter 2). Founded in 1988 the CLC attempts to provide a single voice for over 25,000 construction consultant firms and over 500,000 individual built environment professionals. The vision of the CLC is to be respected and recognised by both the UK construction industry and government as an effective thought leader representing the UK built environment professionals. The CLC has addressed the industry's productivity problem many times, but often with a 'macro' view on the industry as a whole. Both Construction 2025 and The Farmer Review stand firmly behind the CLC, but it could be argued that the CLC leaves the 'micro'-level analysis of the productivity of individual firms and professionals to the professional bodies and research organisations they represent.

10.3 Professional bodies and development requirements in the construction industry

A professional body is an organisation that usually sits within a single profession or part of an industry and consists of individual members that aim to promote best practices and set the standards and expectations of behaviour for both its members and the wider profession. This is often executed by the introduction of codes of conduct and by requiring all members to undertake and record formal and informal professional development. There are many professional bodies operating within the construction industry, and many more than cover professionals both inside and outside of the industry. They all ultimately have the same purpose and similar aims, but specific to the nuanced requirements of their own members. That is the development of their members, through a focus on a development of skill set, experience, and competence. All professional bodies have different requirements. At one end of the scale, this could be a total onus on the individual member to conduct their own development reviews and address any competency deficiencies with no prescription of hours or activity required. At the other end of the scale, it could consist of a fully structured development plan outlining exactly what and for how long a member must participate in designated development opportunities. The most common approach adopted is somewhere in the middle with a specified number of hours to be completed by every member each year on any sort of development activity they feel is required in their professional life and applicable to their professional development needs.

However, despite this professional body focus, there is a lack of research undertaken on the development and productivity of construction sector staff – that which can be considered the 'micro' level. The majority of development and productivity research appears to be focused on the 'macro' level of organisations and industries in general. There is therefore a gap in current understanding with regard to a micro-level analysis of built environment professionals regarding their level of productivity and how this is impacted by their organisation's behaviours. This research seeks to address this gap through surveying the opinions and perceptions of construction professionals through the administration of a questionnaire.

10.4 Research methods

As good practice with all research undertaken to ensure the foundations of the research are in place, a literature review should be conducted to understand the current landscape of the topic in question. Generally, a literature review will help expose any gaps within existing research (Fellows and Liu, 2015) and help serve as a departure point for future explorations within the topic context. In this instance, the contents of this book serve as that literature review, with some of the key arguments and identified gaps in literature summarised in this chapter. One gap that has been revealed in current understandings is around the development perceptions and practices of construction professionals. The research undertaken as part of this book therefore adopts an inductive approach in an attempt to understand the current professional development practices of organisations and what impact this has upon construction professionals. An inductive approach to research is concerned with the generation of theory, often in a data-driven manner deriving from qualitative data that can then be tested (Bell et al., 2018). As this research is exploring a gap in current understanding, the inductive approach adopted will provide a new theory to contribute to concepts and ideas that build on existing knowledge.

As part of this research, questionnaires were distributed to Quantity Surveyors each working for a different construction organisation. Questionnaires are research instruments purposefully designed to yield the required data from each respondent (Babbie, 2016). A questionnaire was selected as the research instrument of choice as it allows for the target audience to be reached and the research completed in a time-effective manner (Bell et al., 2018). Participants also feel a degree of anonymity when completing, therefore allowing for confidential questions to be answered with minimal human contact (Phellas et al., 2012) and perhaps overcoming the potential disadvantage of questions not being answered truthfully (Robson and McCartan, 2017). To help ensure participant understanding of the questionnaire, the questionnaire was presented by the researchers prior to completion by participants and all elements discussed and explained. Attempts to aid participant understanding were also made with the inclusion of mostly closed quantitative questions (Babbie, 2016). The researcher discussions and short closed questions were also used in an attempt to ensure the historically low response rates of questionnaires were improved (Phellas et al., 2012).

Participants were identified and contacted online via email with a request to participate. Thirty-five emails were sent and 24 received positive replies. From the 24 positive replies, 18 questionnaires were eventually completed and returned to the researchers. As each participant was required to work as a Quantity Surveyor, purposive sampling was undertaken whereby each participant was selected for inclusion in the research because they satisfied the research needs (Robson and McCartan, 2017). Once all completed questionnaires were received, the data was compiled and analysed to reveal any patterns and trends.

10.5 Findings and discussion

The results suggest how an organisation approaches the development of its employees has a significant impact upon how the employees approach their own development. Analysis of the questionnaires revealed that 82% of respondents completed some sort of development review with their employer. Out of the 82% who have a development review, 66% see a benefit to development reviews and have some sort of personal development action plan. However, from the 18% of respondents who do not have a work-based development review with their employer, only 20% have any sort of CPD plan in place. The results therefore reveal that an employee is 2.7 times more likely to have a CPD plan in place and take their own professional development seriously if their employer initiates some sort of annual development review (Figure 10.1).

For those who reported that their development review was only held on an annual basis, only 29% felt their employer took the process seriously. This is contrasted with those respondents who reported having a development review with their employer more frequently (every six months, quarterly, and monthly) where 83% reported that they felt their employer took the process seriously. It can therefore be argued that the more frequent regular development reviews are held between employers and employees, the more the likely the employee would feel the employer took the process of their professional development seriously. If an

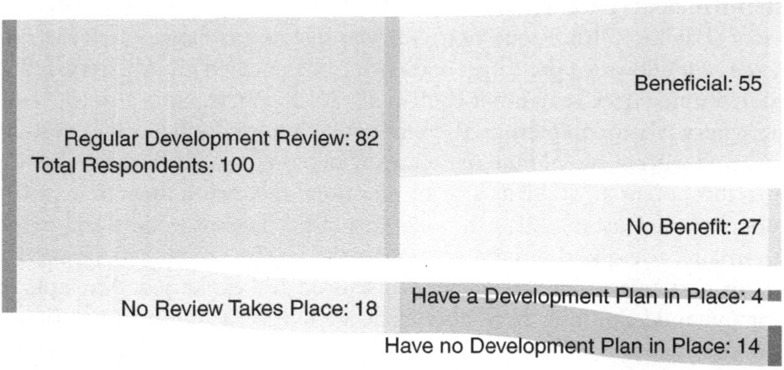

Figure 10.1 Development review results (figures are in percentages).

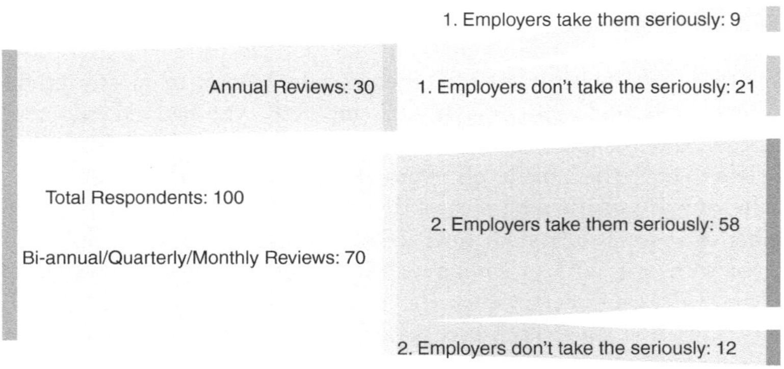

Figure 10.2 Annual and frequent reviews (figures are in percentages).

employer regularly held a development meeting with an employee every month, every quarter, or on a six-month basis, the results reveal the employee would be five times more likely to have a development in place and take their own professional development seriously when compared to an employee whose employer does not hold any development meetings (Figure 10.2).

Further analysis of the results revealed that only 9% of employees took complete control over organising and attending any development training. Thirty-six per cent of employees reported they took joint responsibility along with their employers, and 55% of employees reported that their employers took sole control over their own development through organising any form of development activity. When this is considered in terms of those employees who have development reviews, 64% reported that their development is solely led by their employer and 36% reported that their development is a shared responsibility. Zero per cent of employees who have development reviews reported that they took control of their own development. For those employees who do not have development reviews, 25% reported that they took responsibility for their own development, whilst 50% reported that their development was a shared responsibility with their employer and a further 25% reported that their development opportunities were solely organised by their employers – despite having no form of development review process in place. This could be somewhat worrying as employees who have development reviews from their employers are less likely to take any form of responsibility (either shared with their employer or sole) over their own professional development and instead leave it in the hands of their employers.

Importantly, the results also reveal that 75% of employees whose employer undertook a development review set themselves goals, in the short, medium, or long term. This is compared to only 60% of employees whose employer does not hold some form of development review. Sixty-nine per cent of employees who have a regular development review considered themselves to be 'always' or 'mostly' productive on a weekly basis, whereas only 40% of employees who did not have a regular development review considered themselves to have the same levels of productivity. When this is analysed in further detail, the results reveal that 71% employees who had a regular development review and felt their employer took their development seriously considered themselves to be 'always' or 'mostly' productive on a weekly basis, and again only 40% of employees who had a development review but felt their employer did not take their development seriously considered themselves to have the same levels of productivity.

Finally, analysis of the data reveals that 82% of employees who are currently a member of a professional body have a development review with their employer compared with only 57% of employees who are not members of a professional body. Ninety per cent of employees who are members of a professional body regularly set themselves goals to achieve, again compared with only 57% of those who are not members of a professional body. Fifty-four per cent of employees who are members of a professional body believe their employer takes their development seriously compared to only 14% of those who are not a member of a professional body.

The results therefore indicate that employees who are members of professional bodies and have regular professional development meetings with their employer are more likely to consider their employer to be taking their development seriously. And in turn those employees who feel their employer takes their development seriously are more likely to have a development plan in place, more likely to take or share responsibility of their development, and crucially more likely to consider themselves as productive than both employees who do not have a development review with their employer and those who do have a development review but do not believe their employer takes their development seriously.

10.6 Conclusion

The construction industry is a significant part of the UK economy yet has suffered from what has been described as a 'productivity problem' in that its productivity has remained rather static over the past 50 years when compared to other industries. This problem has been highlighted by many construction reports and addressing it is at the forefront of many current UK government and construction leadership strategies. However, research to date has focused on the productivity of the industry as a whole or at its most detailed upon organisations that operate within it – what can be described as a 'macro' approach. There is a gap in current research around the 'micro' level of productivity analysis – that of built environment professionals themselves. Adopting a questionnaire aimed at Quantity Surveying professionals, this research sought to contribute to this gap in knowledge by understanding the relationship between professional body membership, organisational behaviour, and employee productivity. By understanding current practices, this chapter contributes to an important gap in current research and highlights some important CPD lessons all construction professionals need to be cognisant of. The findings reveal that employees who are members of professional bodies and have regular professional development meetings with their employer are more likely to consider their employer to be taking their development seriously. And in turn those employees who feel their employer takes their development seriously are more likely to have a CPD plan in place, more likely to take or share responsibility for their own development, and crucially more likely to consider themselves as productive when compared to employees who do not have a development review with their employer and employees who do have a development review but do not believe their employer takes their development seriously. This research contributes to current understandings by identifying and contributing to previously unexplored areas of construction productivity research. This research also contributes to the identification of procedures and practices that construction industry organisations may wish to adopt in order to potentially increase the productivity of their workforce. Limitations include the single profession focus and the limited data of 18 questionnaires. In order to confirm any findings, further studies are recommended on different professions within the industry and the use of a wider respondent range where possible.

10.7 References

Babbie, E. (2016). *The Basics of Social Research*. 7th ed. Boston, MA: Cengage Learning.

Bell, E., Bryman, A. and Harley, B. (2018). *Business Research Methods*. 5th ed. Oxford: Oxford University Press.

Carlsson, Bo. (1987). *Productivity Analysis: A Micro-to-Macro Perspective*, IUI Working Paper, No. 181, The Research Institute of Industrial Economics (IUI), Stockholm.

Chartered Institute of Building. (2016). *Productivity in Construction; Creating a Framework for the Industry to Thrive*. Available online at: https://policy.ciob.org/wp-content/uploads/2016/05/CIOB-Productivity-report-2016-v4_single.pdf

Farmer, M. (2016). *The Framer Review of the UK Construction Labour Model; Modernise or Die, Time to Decide the Industry's Future*. Construction Leadership Council.

Fellows, R. and Liu, A. (2015). *Research Methods for Construction*. 4th ed. London: John Wiley and Sons.

Glass, J. and Simmonds, M. (2007). "Considerate construction": Case studies of current practice. *Engineering, Construction and Architectural Management*, 14(2), 131–149.

Office for National Statistics (ONS). (2017). *Construction Output in Great Britain*. Available online at: https://www.ons.gov.uk/businessindustryandtrade/constructionindustry/bulletins/ constructionoutputingreatbritain/

Phellas, C., Bloch, C. and Seale, C. (2012). Structured methods: Interviews, questionnaires and observation. In Seale, C. (Ed) *Researching Society and Culture*. 3rd ed. London: Sage Publications, 182–202.

Rhodes, C. (2019). *Construction Industry: Statistics and Policy*. Nr 01432. House of Commons Library. www.parliament.uk/briefing-papers/sn01432.pdf.

Robson, C. and McCartan, K. (2017). *Real World Research*. 4th ed. London: John Wiley and Sons.

11 Final comments and recommendations for future research

This book has attempted to address a need that exists in the construction industry and a gap that exists in current construction management literature – the continuing professional development (CPD) of construction professionals. The CPD is often an overlooked aspect in the criticism that is levelled at the industry. This criticism is everything from the pollution generated during manufacture and installation to the very methods of construction adopted. The lack of collaboration and the contractual nature of relationships to the reluctance to invest in innovative practices and technology are equally aspects the construction industry is criticised for. This book attempts to pull together these vast criticisms, identify the common construction industry failings, and propose a way forward as to how the industry and professionals operating within it can progress. Namely, this is by the wide-scale adoption of CPD.

Chapter 1 identified what CPD is, the general and widespread benefits it brings to individuals and organisations, and how critical thinking can be adopted to ensure CPD ideas can be aligned with robust and focused career goals. Chapter 2 introduces and explores the construction industry and reports on current CPD practices, identifying the link between the current construction industry issues and the need for CPD to be widely embraced. Chapter 3 then goes on to explore the professional bodies that operate within the construction industry, their purpose, entry requirements, and how each focuses upon the CPD of members. Chapter 4 then outlines how and why goals should be set as part of a CPD plan and discusses the tools and mechanisms that can be employed to set goals that have an increased chance of being successful achieved. Chapter 5 builds on these goals set by illustrating how and why CPD plans should be developed around these goals so that milestones to success can be identified and progress can be monitored and recorded to aid motivation and also allow progress to be shared if required. Chapter 6 discusses the skills required to reflect upon CPD progress. Learning modules are introduced, as are reflective models, both serving to support individuals in becoming reflective practitioners. Chapter 7 highlights and tackles the issues of organisations and CPD, which can prove to be especially problematic in the somewhat temporary nature of the construction industry organisation. Human resource management in regard to career development is also included as is how this links to the requirements and offerings of construction industry professional bodies. Chapter 8 discusses how the CPD of others can be effectively managed and it aimed at individuals within construction organisations who have line management responsibility for the professional development of others. The role of mentoring and the benefits it provides for all concerned in increasing and improving skill sets are also discussed. Chapter 9 utilises examples of development initiatives from both inside and outside of the construction industry. Chapter 10 attempts to pull some of the literature covered in these chapters together and discusses the 'productivity problem' the construction introduces faces. Questionnaire-based research and analysis of the completed responses reveal the positive impacts professional bodies and organisations that focus on CPD can have on individual employees' development, motivation, and productivity.

Based on the topics, ideas, and concepts discussed in this book, as well as the original research undertaken, to move the research agenda forward for CPD in the built environment, the following research directions for future research are proposed:

1. The construction industry needs to address the common and underlying issues across several reports in that it is the skill sets of the construction professionals tasked to deliver the changes required that is of the upmost importance in successfully meeting future challenges and demands.
2. The 'micro level' of construction productivity needs to be explored. The 'macro level' of the industry as a whole shows that the construction industry suffers from a 'productivity problem', but there is a lack of research and understanding about the 'micro level' of construction professionals' individual productivity.
3. Case studies of construction organisations need to be developed to contrast and compare the approaches currently undertaken towards professional development of employees, and how this differs from small, medium, and large organisations, and the differences experienced by organisations between those that invest in their employees' professional development and those that do not.
4. Research is required into the benefits of CPD behaviour and how, as a mechanism for increasing skill sets, CPD can be utilised on a larger scale to tackle the issues currently facing the industry,
5. Professional bodies need to collaborate and share the data they have on members' professional development. This will help enable an industry best practice model to be established, where successful CPD practices can be built upon and unsuccessful practices can be identified and eliminated to ensure all construction organisations and professionals who engage CPD do so successfully.
6. CPD practices need to be widely rolled out as part of the education of construction professionals, at all levels of educational systems, so the benefits can be experienced and best practices can be built upon and adopted over a longer period of time.

Index

Note: **Bold** page numbers refer to tables and *italic* page numbers refer to figures.